JUST AS MUCH A WOMAN

To Olga and Yuri,
With love -
Nancy

Also by Nancy Rosenfeld
Unfinished Journey: "From Tyranny to Freedom"

Nancy Rosenfeld
and
Dianna W. Bolen, Psy.D

JUST AS MUCH A WOMAN

YOUR PERSONAL GUIDE TO HYSTERECTOMY AND BEYOND

Prima Publishing

Illustrations by Scott Wills.

Library of Congress Cataloging-in-Publication Data on File

99 00 01 02 03 HH 10 9 8 7 6 5 4 3 2 1
Printed in the United States of America

How to Order
Single copies may be ordered from Prima Publishing, P.O. Box 1260BK, Rocklin, CA 95677; telephone (916) 632-4400. Quantity discounts are also available. On your letterhead, include information concerning the intended use of the books and the number of books you wish to purchase.

Visit us online at *www.primalife.com*

To Marty, my best friend and life partner,
who has supported my work with
unfailing patience and love.

—Nancy Rosenfeld

To my mother, Virginia Kowalski,
who died of ovarian cancer in 1993.
Her characteristics of determination
and abundant love have been
a source of strength in me.

—Dianna W. Bolen

CONTENTS

ACKNOWLEDGMENTS

THE WRITING of this book was a team effort and could not have been accomplished without the dedicated help and support of everyone involved.

At the heart of the book is the contribution made by all those women who unselfishly gave of themselves by candidly revealing their personal stories for the benefit of our research. It is to them whom we remain most deeply grateful and humbled.

With love and gratitude I also want to thank my husband Marty, whose unwavering patience and understanding for more than one year sustained me while I remained driven to complete the manuscript. Without his love it would have been difficult to attain the necessary strength required to finish a book of this magnitude.

Coauthor Dianna Bolen offered invaluable assistance through her extraordinary skill, keen insight, and dauntless commitment to our project. She became a dedicated partner in every phase of our mutual endeavor. Dianna's professional knowledge and sensitivity, along with her uncanny ability to both hear and see what was taking place behind the scenes of every action, both amazed and inspired me. Not only was she right on target every time with advice, but she worked hard at finding just the right word to convey the intended meaning of any particular sentence or episode. In addition, Dianna gave me added encouragement and confidence by introducing me to other professionals whose services proved essential for the success of this undertaking as a whole.

After Dianna's and my work on the manuscript had finally been completed, we then turned it over to the next member of our team, Sharon Ozimek. Sharon, a copy editor, was given the awesome task of shaping our manuscript into proper structural and grammatical form for submission for publication.

Our deepest respect and appreciation go to the team of doctors who generously gave of their time to proofread the manuscript for any medical errors and inconsistencies: Dr. Martin Kass, my gynecologist for more than twelve years and the doctor who performed my hysterectomy; Dr. Harry Burstein, chairman of the Department of Obstetrics and Gynecology at Highland Park Hospital and the one called in to assist with my surgery; and Dr. Heather Krantz, an associate of Dr. Kass and Dr. Burstein.

Scott Wills worked painstakingly hard at illustrating our manuscript with medically accurate and original drawings. He patiently worked with Dianna and me by sketching figures and diagrams from different perspectives before achieving the correct interpretation.

Ruyell Ho, a professional painter and photographer, donated his services by offering to give both Dianna and me a photographic session. His beautiful portrait of the two of us appears on the book jacket.

Hazel Gitlitz, owner and president of the Multiplex Health and Fitness Center, helped organize the women's workshop while providing an ideal setting for it to take place. The findings from the workshop have also been documented in the book.

Dr. Sebastian Faro, the distinguished professor and chairman of the Department of Obstetrics and Gynecology at Rush-Presbyterian-St. Luke's Medical Center, Chicago, accepted our request to write the foreword to this book. Dr. Faro, who has authored several books on obstetrics and gynecology, is also editor in chief of a bimonthly medical journal on infectious diseases. He graciously arranged to meet with Dianna and me in the middle of his hectic schedule, sandwiching us in between surgery and medical conferences overseas.

A very special thanks to my wonderful son, Stephen Rosenfeld, who donated his services by agreeing to do all of our legal work free of charge.

Finally, our most sincere appreciation to the staff at Prima Publishing for their enthusiastic response and professional acumen: Jamie Miller, acquisition editor, whose job was to oversee the entire project from beginning to end; Steven Bratman, M.D., medical editor, who examined the manuscript for medical accuracy; Jennifer Fox and Laura Larson, who did a yeoman's job as copy editors; and publisher Ben Dominitz, who brainstormed our new title, *Just As Much a Woman*. That was the decisive moment when we knew we had found the right house! Ben had immediately understood the essence of our book, a feat not easily attainable for a man when dealing with a "woman's only" issue.

—Nancy Rosenfeld

I HAVE been avoiding the task of writing the acknowledgments because it signifies the end of a project that has been the inspiration for intensive efforts on the part of many dedicated and talented people. With this project's ending comes the "letting go" of the opportunity to make one last change, to add one last thought. It also means the dissolution of our "team." Despite my feelings of finality, I am also aware of the tremendous gifts I have received by being invited to become a part of this project. I have been privileged to work alongside all of these dedicated and talented people, and I have learned just how valuable my personal support system is to me.

It was Nancy's vision and commitment that gave birth to this book and enabled it to be written. But it was also Nancy's openness to my probing queries and her receptiveness to my direct and candid feedback that allowed us to enrich that vision and deepen the commitment to providing the best possible resource for you, the reader.

I am deeply grateful to Sharon Ozimek, who has been my trusted and deeply respected editor for many years. Sharon possesses a phenomenal ability to identify and clearly communicate needed changes. She is both patient and relentless in her pursuit of quality.

I am also grateful to Ruyell Ho for his keen abilities and visual aesthetic judgment in the creation of the photographs he made for us to be used in the promotion of this book. Thanks also to Scott Wills, an author in his own right, who provided the pencil sketches that illustrate this manuscript. Scott also provided helpful hints about becoming published.

Finally, I want to thank all of those people who clearly and unfailingly supported me regardless of whether they understood my struggles or shared my vision. Several of these people deserve special mention. I want to express my gratitude to my cousin Gene Hamilton and my dear friends James Unland, Ernie Klemme, and John and Iriss Blaine.

—Dianna W. Bolen

FOREWORD

EVERY WOMAN who must undergo surgery faces fear and, to a degree, concern regarding the change it may necessitate in her lifestyle. Most women have surgery because of either a malfunctioning organ or one that is diseased and needs to be corrected or removed. The organ abnormality either impedes the patient's health or may be seriously placing her life in jeopardy. Initially, the greatest concern is whether or not she will survive the operative procedure. The expectation is that all will be well, and she will be able to resume or improve her life. Most often, the result of the operative procedure will not impart a long-lasting significant change in her life.

However, the woman undergoing a hysterectomy faces uncertainties that other surgery patients do not. The reason for the hysterectomy, in most instances, is not because the condition is life threatening, but because quality of life is suffering. Nancy Rosenfeld and Dianna Bolen bring the reality of the entire process of a hysterectomy to life in their book. They explain what it actually means to be told that a hysterectomy is indicated, and they address the confusion that often arises when a second opinion is obtained. They detail the fears that a patient is confronted with when a hysterectomy is needed, the thoughts that surface when thinking about the operative procedure, and the interaction that occurs with various individuals including health care providers, family, and friends. This book contains extremely important events in the chronology of a patient undergoing a hysterectomy, including the emptiness that some women experience and the freedom expressed by others.

The spectrum of feelings and concerns revealed by both Nancy and the patients she interviewed makes an extremely informative journal, which must be read by both practicing obstetricians and gynecologists as well as young physicians in training in order to understand the importance of proper communication between the physician and the patient. Nancy comfortably brings to light the important role that the physician plays in mentally preparing the patient for surgery, not just at the time when a hysterectomy is indicated, but also when any potential problems are discovered.

The physician should educate the patient throughout the time medical care is rendered, and this book will serve as an important part of that preparation. After the initial discussion, the patient must assume the responsibility of researching the subject. This is necessary so she can ask questions and ensure that she is knowledgeable about the operation and the consequences of the surgery. I recommend that *all* physicians, not just gynecologists, urge their patients with gynecological problems to read this book. It is a book for all women who may require a hysterectomy now or in the future. The book's recommendations for mentally and physically preparing for a hysterectomy are excellent, the posthysterectomy suggestions are solid, and the descriptions of complications are addressed with frank honesty. This is another excellent point for physicians and nurses to note, as detailed preoperative discussion of the potential complications and what is to be expected in the immediate postoperative period might hasten the patient's recovery.

Dianna brings directly into focus one area that is often poorly addressed by physicians: sex. Most couples are usually very concerned about their sexual life following the hysterectomy. This is an extremely important subject that is dealt with openly by both the authors and the interviewed patients. The authors also point out the importance of honesty within oneself regarding the degree of satisfaction in the sexual relationship. This, in conjunction with the physician openly discussing what is to be expected following surgery, will help the patient to adjust to any change that may occur. The helpfulness of this section to physicians and patients cannot be overstated.

It is also important for the physician to discuss lifetime care with the patient. Unlike most surgical procedures, a hysterectomy is usually performed on women who are healthy. However, following surgery these otherwise healthy women need long-term medical follow-up. The authors, again, bring this to the forefront, pointing out that follow-up care should include discussions about hormonal replacement, breast cancer, osteoporosis, heart disease, and memory loss. Because nurses play a significant role in providing this care, I would also recommend that they read this book. It should be noted that a female nurse or physician who has not had a hysterectomy does not have any more of an understanding of what the patient is experiencing than a male physician or nurse does.

In addition, I recommend that members of the patient's family, especially the partner, read this book. All too often those who are not experiencing the operation cannot possibly understand the trauma that the patient is facing. Women who have had a hysterectomy need support, most importantly during the immediate periods preceding and following the operation, and then for several months thereafter to adjust to the change that the procedure has caused in their bodies. I further recommend that employers, both men and women, read this book to develop a better understanding of how a hysterectomy might affect an employee.

The problems that a hysterectomy raises are not minor and should not be minimized for they create a lifetime of concerns. I commend Nancy's frank truthfulness and her taking this personal experience public to allow women to benefit not only from her story but from the stories of other women as well.

—*Sebastian Faro,* M.D., Ph.D.
John M. Simpson Professor and Chairman
Department of Obstetrics and Gynecology
Rush-Presbyterian-St. Luke's Medical Center
Chicago, Illinois

INTRODUCTION

THE BIRTH of this book occurred, most fittingly, in a hospital on the very day of surgery. It was then that I resolved to document my story.

Like many others who have never experienced major surgery, I was filled with anxiety. So many uncertainties lay ahead. The loss of control after being anesthetized was an issue, not to mention the operation itself. Yet, there were deeper reasons for my uneasiness, the most disturbing of which regarded questions dealing with lost youth, femininity, and sexuality.

Prior to being operated on, I canvassed book stores and libraries for material concerning my particular medical condition and what lay ahead. What I discovered on the subject of hysterectomies was, unfortunately, limited and often negative. I read scores of case histories—women relating their horror stories. Yet if a hysterectomy was something feared by so many, and if the lives of hysterectomized women were permanently damaged, why then were so many surgical procedures being performed annually?

I nevertheless had faith in my doctor's recommendation. However, before agreeing to have surgery I consulted with two other physicians—the family doctor and another gynecologist. Both concurred that it was a "no-choice" situation.

My reason for writing this book was to explore hysterectomies from the vantage point of a patient, a woman. I had traveled that road of fear, anxiety, and uncertainty and then discovered an alternate route.

I began to gather information on the subject of hysterectomy, first by conducting an intensive search for books and medical journals. During this investigation professionals in the field were frequently consulted. I also interviewed countless women, some of whom were also struggling with surgery-related problems and issues. Many of their stories were inspirational, and I found that I could empathize, as one girlfriend to another, inasmuch as I had walked the same path. Eventually, a support group (or women's forum) was formed to help hysterectomized women resolve many of the issues we all faced following surgery.

Knowledge provides the basic map for understanding and conquering our fear; *humor* is our ability to enjoy the scenery along the journey. All of us during our lifetime cross many roads and bridges, sometimes losing our direction and finding no way back. Having come to the end of a road, we may feel blocked, anxious, or frightened. Although we may know it's important to move on, at times there is so much uncertainty as to just *where* that new road lies.

This book contains medically correct and detailed information about hysterectomy suitable for the layperson. In addition, it outlines the stages of the hysterectomy process from diagnosis to recovery, both physically and emotionally. It also provides an introspective and sometimes humorous personal narrative of the experience as well as delving into cases of others. I was especially drawn to some of the women whom you will meet in this book. The poignancy of their stories is deeply moving, sometimes painfully so, yet always inspirational.

One year from the time I first embarked on this writing assignment and was completing the first draft of the manuscript, I had a meeting with Dianna Bolen. Dianna, a researcher and licensed psychotherapist, had compiled all of the statistical data from a questionnaire survey that had been conducted as part of the research for this book. She had also led the fifth session of the women's workshop. At this point we decided to join forces and work together on the manuscript. As coauthor of this venture, Dianna would serve as a consultant and chief editor as well as joining me in all aspects regarding the undertaking of this endeavor.

What I could never have envisioned is the inspirational quality of Dianna's work. She became my alter ego. When I conveyed to her what I was doing in any particular passage, she told me what I was thinking and the reasons behind my actions. And she was right, consistently! Together, we became an energizing force of stimulation and creativity for each other—a dynamic duo.

This is a book to help you find your right path from among the alternatives before you. I'm confident that once you do discover it, your own inspiration will follow. *Just As Much a Woman* is the book I needed to find before my own surgery, but it wasn't out there.

—Nancy Rosenfeld

JUST AS MUCH A WOMAN

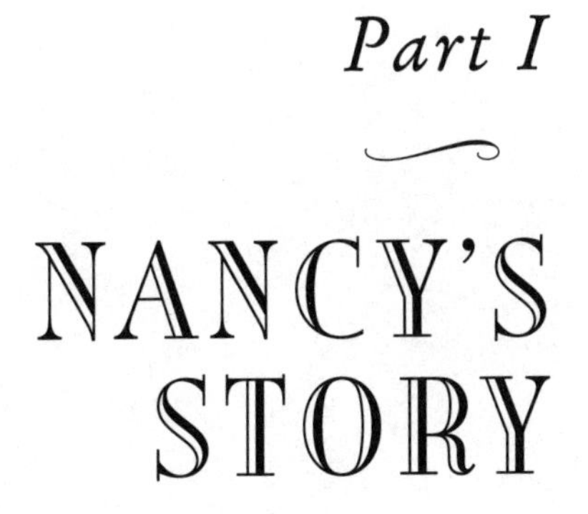

Part I

NANCY'S STORY

CHAPTER ONE

DISCOVERY

WITHOUT WARNING, I came face to face with my own mortality in the spring of 1996. It hit me at a time when I was feeling newly restored and at peace, a period of happiness and tranquility and of summer plans that held great promise. Following years of trial and unrest, I had just rediscovered *la joie de vie*.

Then, suddenly, something happened that threatened to rock the boat—jeopardizing not only my personal security and well-being but my very self-image. It was not something unspeakably horrible, nor was it the greatest misfortune ever to befall my life.

At some point, everyone is confronted with the reality of passing time when we see those around us begin to fade and weaken. This awareness does not happen overnight but is a gradual evolution over time. Seldom, in fact, do we see ourselves aging but are nevertheless shocked by the decay we find in others—for example, when we meet former classmates whom we haven't seen in years: the beautiful cheerleader turned matronly; the football hero, now fat and bald. Oh, my God! What happened?

Sooner or later when the security blanket of youth gets blown away, we come to grips with the realization that none of us is immune to loss. Marriages break apart; dreams go up in smoke; we become empty nesters; health, once taken for granted, begins to fail, and parents grow old and infirm. None of us can escape life's only two certainties: uncertainty and death.

My awakening, which caused me great anxiety, was kindled by the sudden and unexpected emergence of a new fork in the road—a turning point, the passage from one stage of life to another, a loss.

I had gone for my regular six-month checkup. Nothing was wrong; I felt fine. Dr. Kass, my gynecologist, was his usual friendly self, always appearing to be genuinely interested in his patients so that there was never a moment of discomfort during a routine exam. He had even surprised me a few years earlier by attending a book signing following the publication of my first book.

Nothing unusual differentiated this exam from prior checkups. After he finished, I was told to get dressed and come into his office, the same as always. When I walked in, he greeted me in his usual pleasant manner.

"Sit down, Nancy," he said "but you may wish to first close the door." Without giving it a second thought I followed his suggestion. "I see in my records," he continued, "that it's been over a year since your last mammogram. I know you shy away from them, but perhaps I may give you some incentive to make that appointment soon."

"Why?" I asked, detecting the serious tone of his voice, although his facial expression remained noncommittal.

"Because you might kill two birds with one stone," he said, "by taking an ultrasound at the time of your mammogram." Pausing for a moment, he went on. "You have what I believe to be a benign fibroid tumor on the back wall of the uterus."

"A what?" I asked, focusing only on the word *tumor.*

"A nonmalignant fibroid tumor," he slowly repeated, carefully emphasizing *nonmalignant.* "It's common for women to have fibroids, and many times they disappear by themselves when left alone. Especially when a woman enters menopause these fibroids tend to shrink in size and go away naturally, so there's no need for surgery. But," he paused, "in your case I would recommend taking it out because of its size and the fact that you're not yet menopausal."

"But why? How big is it?" I pressed, feeling a growing sense of uneasiness.

"About the size of a grapefruit."

"A grapefruit?" I gasped. "I can't believe it! What if it *is* cancerous? Why haven't I noticed it? Why . . . ?"

"Don't worry!" he quickly interjected. "Fibroids are almost never malignant, and as far as the size, don't you realize how much thinner you'd be without all that thickness around your belly?" Though it hadn't occurred to me before, now I did think about how difficult it had seemed to remain on the light side of 120 pounds. Although that may be hardly obese for a woman five feet, four inches tall, it was still an increase of several pounds over the past year.

Today a hysterectomy may be regarded as common surgery, but for me it signaled something far more onerous—that undeniable stage called "midlife," the crossroads from youth to maturity and of facing up to one's own mortality.

"No," I admitted, truthfully. "I hadn't realized. But what type of surgery are you talking about?"

"A complete hysterectomy."

"A complete whaaaat?" I stammered, my anxiety sharply escalating. "But, I've never had anything more serious than a tonsillectomy or broken wrist. If I have a hysterectomy, I'll go right into menopause."

"That's right, but that's my recommendation," Dr. Kass continued. "We can put you on hormone therapy or herbal treatments right after surgery to help replenish your natural supply of hormones. Believe me—you'll be fine."

I felt my panic rising. I may have passed the big five-oh, but I wasn't ready for this. Today a hysterectomy may be regarded as common surgery, but for me it signaled something far more onerous—that undeniable stage called "midlife," the crossroads from youth to maturity and of facing up to one's own mortality. The feeling of no longer being regarded as young and vital, but "older," on the road to becoming a senior citizen, the nonstop ticking of the clock.

"But," I continued, "won't a complete hysterectomy make me look and feel older because I'll lose my female hormones? Isn't it true that after a woman's ovaries stop functioning the aging process begins immediately? And what about my skin? And my weight? And what about the feeling of being castrated—the loss of my femininity and sexuality?"

As my thoughts trailed off, Dr. Kass listened patiently to my rattling on and on about my vain concerns, displaying no sign of intolerance but instead flashing a warm, gentle smile.

"Nancy," he offered reassuringly, "everything will be fine. Trust me. Nothing will happen to you, I promise. You won't look any different, but you'll feel a whole lot better. We can start you on estrogen. Hormone replacement therapy (HRT) also prevents osteoporosis, heart disease, and other problems associated with menopause. Although there may be relative contraindications (conditions indicating against the advisability of a particular treatment), the only *absolute* contraindications are (1) active thrombophlebitis (blood clots) and (2) the recent incidence of breast or uterine cancer. Sometimes, women with cystic breasts are advised against it. However, each case must be treated on an individual basis, besides which you don't fall into these categories and I *can* prescribe estrogen for you."

Still not ready to accept the situation, I tried bargaining.

"Can't you take out the tumor but leave my ovaries alone?" I begged. "Especially if they're healthy?"

"You don't need them anymore," he insisted. "You're not going to have more children, and we don't want to run the risk of ovarian cancer. It could happen later on, and ovarian cancer is dangerous." He paused to make certain I was listening. "This way, we're taking no chances and avoiding any possibility of future surgery."

While staring into space, I was slowly digesting the new turn of events. I responded flatly, "Is this something that must be done right away, or can it wait?"

"It's *not* an emergency," he said quickly, "but I still want you to have the ultrasound and mammogram right away. Then we'll go from there."

"How about September?" I quizzed, trying to regain my optimism.

"There's no reason why not," he said. "Let's just wait and see how everything looks on the ultrasound. If it's what I think, we'll monitor your condition every three weeks from now until September. As long as there's no significant change, early September should be OK. But no longer," he warned.

Though Dr. Kass did everything possible to allay my fears, I was filled with anxiety after leaving his office. Never having had major surgery, this news was a shock. Furthermore, whether or not I was interested in bearing more children didn't eliminate the fear of potential loss. Because female reproduction represents the very essence of womanhood, would my feminine self-image suffer after removal of these vital parts?

For the remainder of the day I lost all ability to concentrate on anything but fibroid tumors and hysterectomies. I drove into town and walked around in a daze. When I came home I ran into the bathroom to examine my stomach in the full-length mirror. Sure

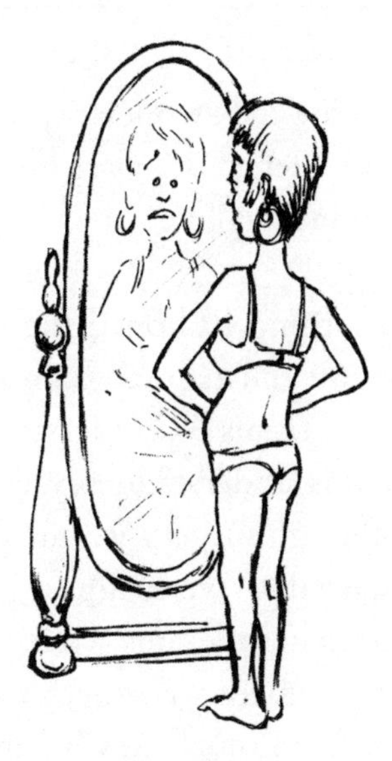

TERMS TO UNDERSTAND

Hysterectomy—Approximately 590,000 hysterectomies are performed every year in the United States. Hysterectomies rank as the second most frequently performed major surgery for women in this country (cesarean section is first). Although total hysterectomy rates among African-American women are similar to those for Caucasian women, African Americans seem to be more prone to develop fibroids than Caucasian women. Moreover, African-American patients tend to be younger.[1]

Magnetic resonance imaging (MRI)—An MRI, also known as *nuclear magnetic resonance,* is a procedure for diagnosing disorders based on the electrical resonance within the body.[2]

Mammogram—A mammogram, which is a diagnostic X-ray of the breast, is a screening technique that can detect some cancers before they are felt. This procedure is recommended on an annual basis for women over fifty as well as younger women who fall into a high-risk group.[3]

Menopause—Menopause is defined as the "change of life" or the final "pause" of menstruation. When it occurs normally rather than surgically, a gradual slowing down and irregularity of the menstrual cycle occur before the actual cessation of menstruation.

enough—my abdomen looked swollen. I pressed my stomach and thought I could not only detect the mass but also see it protruding from behind the abdominal wall.

THE FOLLOWING morning I phoned the radiology department of the hospital to schedule the mammogram and ultrasound for the next week (see the box "Terms to Understand" and the glossary). My husband, Marty, was understandably concerned when I first gave him the news, although surgery was nothing new to him since he himself had experienced it several times.

My concern about mammograms was soon put to rest when I discovered the new equipment that the hospital had recently installed made the procedure much less uncomfortable. The nurse

Ultrasound—An ultrasound is a picture (or sonogram) of internal organs through the use of sound waves. A small, wandlike instrument, waved over the examining parts, sends sound waves to the organs that are then transmitted and reflected onto a monitor.[4]

Uterine fibroid tumors—Fibroid tumors are benign (noncancerous) tumors composed of fibrous, fatty tissue that stem from the smooth muscle cells of the uterus. Also called *uterine myoma,* these benign muscle tumors are very common, occurring in 20 percent of all women.[5] Frequently they are found in clusters rather than a single fibroid. When small and posing no problems, they can be left alone and sometimes may even dissolve naturally. However, when these fibroids enlarge, they can interfere with surrounding organs and other vital tissue, such as the bladder and intestines, by pressing against them and pushing them out of position. Noticeable symptoms that might indicate surgery are bloating, pain, and bleeding. A more detailed discussion of fibroids appears in the next chapter.

urged me to relax because the machine no longer compressed the breast with the same amount of pressure. It had been customary to use twenty-five pounds of pressure in compressing breast tissue, and that hurt. Now, however, health professionals have discovered they can obtain an accurate reading with a minimum of just five pounds of pressure, which makes the procedure almost painless. I told the nurse about an earlier experience when the pain from the mammogram had been so intense that I had fainted. She wasn't surprised.

Men don't always understand the discomfort involved with having a mammogram. Once I informed Dr. Kass how I felt about taking them. "How would you feel," I had asked him, "if someone took your private parts and compressed them down to the size of a pancake?" "I know," he had responded with a very straight face, "and you're not the first one to make the comparison."

Before having an ultrasound, you need to have a full bladder so you must drink several glasses of water ahead of time. The test itself is comfortable, but the pressure on your belly from the scanning equipment makes you feel like you need to urinate.

My technician, a pleasant young woman, took several pictures of my abdominal area in an effort to get a good look at the uterus and ovaries. However, no matter how hard she tried to get a sharp picture, the image appeared very gray and fuzzy on the screen. I, too, could see the screen from where I was positioned on the table. When it is difficult to get a sharp reading on the monitor, as it was in my case, an intravaginal probe may also be required.

At last the procedure was over. The technician told me that although the images still appeared fuzzy, the radiologist would be able to see clearly enough to make a proper diagnosis. Within twenty-four hours Dr. Kass would have the radiology report, and I could phone him for the results.

The findings of the radiology report coincided with Dr. Kass's expectations and stated the following:

> The uterus demonstrates a large hypo echoic mass growing off the posterior aspect of the fundus and body of the uterus measuring over 6 cm in diameter. This probably represents a large fibroid. There appears to be a small cervical cyst. The right ovary demonstrates a somewhat lobulated hypo to anechoic rounded structure associated with it measuring close to 15 mm in diameter, probably representing a small cyst or dominant follicle. It doesn't meet the strict criteria for a simple cyst because it is not round and does not have a smooth wall. The left ovary is not as well seen but no left adnexal mass is identified. IMPRESSION: There is a large pelvic mass that is immediately contiguous with the posterior aspect of the uterus and I think this probably represents a large fibroid.

After receiving the radiology report, I telephoned my internist to give him the news and seek his advice. He suggested a consultation with a second physician because there may be alternatives to surgery or, perhaps, other types of surgery better suited to an individual patient's condition. Most conscientious doctors welcome another opinion, and some hospitals even *insist* on it.

If you don't know of another doctor to consult for a second opinion, ask your insurance company for recommendations or call the American Medical Association (AMA). Also check with your insurance company about covered medical services, as well as limitations on coverage and its requirements.

A typical requirement of many insurance companies is obtaining precertification for your admission. Precertification ensures that your insurance will pay the agreed-on portion of your bill.

This time my internist also felt that more than one additional opinion would be superfluous because second and third opinions are often more radical. I received the name of a prominent physician who specialized in oncology/gynecology. With his advice, I felt I'd need no other. Yet, his was such a busy practice that I was obliged to wait three and a half weeks for an appointment.

I maintained my usual busy schedule, trying not to concentrate on my medical condition. I was working three days a week, swam almost daily at the health club, worked out in the gym, and kept a busy social calendar. I also went in search of all available information on fibroid tumors and hysterectomies by checking out the local bookstores and library. I was filled with questions and concerns; I needed answers.

If the surgery is not urgent or mandatory, a woman who does her homework will discover both surgical and nonsurgical options.

A hysterectomy (see the box "Terms to Understand" and the glossary) is a serious procedure because it involves major abdominal surgery and poses certain risks. Nevertheless, it rarely endangers a patient's life unless she already has serious health problems. In these cases the physician may opt to avoid surgery entirely. Experts in the field cite specific reasons that a woman should undergo the operation. Justification for surgery includes uterine cancer, a precancerous condition, large fibroid tumors, and uncontrollable bleeding. Yet, even when a hysterectomy has been recommended, it is rarely an emergency situation requiring immediate surgery. Only in those cases involving excessive bleeding, constant pain, or the likelihood of cancer would surgery be mandatory without further delay.

A great majority of women do have the luxury of postponing surgery and should take the time to explore their options. If the surgery is not urgent or mandatory, a woman who does her homework will discover both surgical and nonsurgical options. She should then carefully weigh possible alternatives and discuss them with her physician before making a final decision. But first, a woman must face reality and be willing to accept that *a problem exists* that will not disappear.

COAUTHOR DIANNA BOLEN believes this task of facing reality is usually a difficult and stressful undertaking. Women vary in their ability to face adversity, depending on their personality. For example, an easygoing person may not be assertive enough to ensure her own proper care, and a perfectionist may postpone her decision far too long because she feels she lacks information. A person who is prone to deny problems may turn to drugs, alcohol, food, or television as a means of escape. Other differences in facing adversity have to do with prior life experiences.

A woman who has been making important decisions for most of her life is much better prepared for the decisions associated with hysterectomy than someone who has had most of her decisions made for her, perhaps as a result of deferring to another (i.e., a husband, parent, friend, or relative). Also, recent and life-long stressors play an active role. For example, a woman who has struggled all her life for simple necessities such as food and shelter may feel depleted and unable to cope with additional problems. A woman who has recently lost a loved one, through death or divorce, or who lacks adequate social supports may say to herself, "What now?" Women with disabilities, mental illness, or low intelligence are also not exempt from the difficulty of making decisions regarding hysterectomy.

"No matter what your lot in life," says Dianna, "you will be required to draw upon whatever resources you have and to reach out, and to reach from within, for new resources to deal with this challenging life experience." The actual fact-finding process is a way to help a woman accept reality so she can go forward and make that right decision. It is a way to become gradually acclimated to the idea of surgery and to become an informed consumer.

Libraries are available to everyone. Dianna suggests that you start with simple, easy-to-understand information. If you find yourself becoming anxious or experiencing difficulty concentrating, Dianna advises that you set a manageable goal such as reading four pages or making a list of questions for your doctor. Then, reward yourself for attaining that goal.

Your active participation in decisions regarding your hysterectomy is essential. However, you must have information before you can make an informed decision. Making informed decisions is empowering. Women who do avail themselves of the opportunity to participate in decisions regarding their health care are likely to feel more comfortable with their ultimate decision to have or not to have a hysterectomy. On the other hand, if you permit others to take over your responsibilities, you may feel victimized and suffer lifelong regrets.

Another reason for delaying surgery is to give you time to improve your health and fitness. Combining daily exercise, proper rest, good nutritional habits, a well-balanced diet, plus supplementary daily vitamins will help shorten the recovery period while improving your overall health. Breathing exercises will also help you relax at the time of surgery as well as help ease the pain afterward.

Finally, that most pressing question for most women: *Will a hysterectomy affect my feelings of femininity?* When I was contemplating my choices, I sat down with pencil and paper and listed the pluses and minuses regarding surgery. On my plus list:

1. Threats of cancer eliminated
2. No more pain and swelling due to fibroid growth
3. Permanent cessation of menstruation

4. Elimination of spotting that causes embarrassing clothing stains
5. Freedom of vacationing without bothering with menstrual cycle
6. Elimination of bloating, swelling, and skin eruptions common to menstruation
7. Permanent infertility, eliminating need for contraception

Next, the minuses:

1. The feeling of being castrated or neutered
2. Possible diminished sexual drive
3. Hot flashes and premature aging

First, the fear of losing one's femininity from castration is an erroneous assumption because a woman's libido does not exist in her erogenous zones but rather in her brain. Physical changes, however, affecting a woman's sexuality do occur but are frequently undetected. Finally, hot flashes and premature aging (after removal of ovaries) *can* be controlled by estrogen with the use of hormone replacement therapy (HRT).

Premature aging was nevertheless my greatest anxiety prior to surgery because I so clearly remember a friend's experience eight years earlier. Despite the fact that hers was a vaginal hysterectomy rather than abdominal, she commented that in the hospital she had felt totally miserable and unattractive after surgery. "But my ovaries were not removed," she exclaimed, "so I won't experience menopause for years. Menopause turns women into old ladies, and their skin gets dry and wrinkled and starts to sag." Her remarks returned to haunt me when I learned of my own need to undergo surgery. The result: I felt compelled to avoid "instant aging" at all costs if that was, in fact, what happened with menopause (see the box and glossary). However, because decreasing levels of estrogen are responsible for problems such as thinning and drying of vaginal and urinary tissues and aging skin, a supplementary dosage of estrogen can help counteract the problems associated with menopause.

Before the onset of menopause is a seven-year transitional period called the *perimenopausal* stage. Perimenopause usually begins anytime after a woman enters her forties and can continue through her middle fifties. During this time there is a gradual decrease in the levels of estrogen and progesterone. Both estrogen and progesterone are produced by the ovaries as well as by the adrenal glands (located near the kidneys).

Symptoms experienced by women going through menopause include hot flashes (or flushes), night sweats, vaginal dryness and soreness during sexual intercourse, irritability, insomnia, headaches, incontinence, weight gain, fatigue, depression, and backaches. HRT can help alleviate these uncomfortable symptoms by resupplying the body with the missing hormones.

THE FOLLOWING week Marty accompanied me on my visit to the specialist. Neither Marty nor I felt terribly concerned about what the doctor might say. We assumed his opinion would not differ sharply from Dr. Kass's.

Looking at Marty now, he appeared so dapper. Tall, well built, and very handsome, he was dressed in a light brown suit and was sporting a new, flamboyant tie with coordinated pocket square—his trademark. The color of his suit went well with his ruddy complexion and thick brown hair, now slightly salted. How lucky I was to have a husband like him! How many times have I taken Marty for granted, I pondered? Like most husbands and wives we've had our petty squabbles, and yet regardless of our differences I appreciated his now being by my side. I was not alone.

"Well, Nancy," the doctor began, "I must be honest. You do have a large uterine tumor, but I'm not sure it's a fibroid. It could be malignant. I'd say you have a sixty/forty chance of it not being cancerous."

"What?" I stammered, feeling suddenly shocked and short of breath. "But I thought the ultrasound test proved it's a benign fibroid."

"No," said the doctor. "An ultrasound can only determine that there's a definite mass, but we cannot tell for certain what kind of a mass. It could be a fibroid, but it could also be a malignant tumor."

I felt panicky as I stared at Marty, searching for his reaction. His face looked ashen.

"What are you telling me? What do you think I should do?"

"I think you should check into the hospital immediately for surgery this week. You don't want to fool around with something like this."

"I can't," I responded, vehemently refusing to believe what I had just heard. "I'm busy because we have friends in town from out of the country. If you still feel I have better than a fifty-fifty chance, then what alternatives do I have?"

"Nancy!" said Marty. "Think about what you're saying. Nothing is more important than your health. If you need surgery now, our friends will come to the hospital."

"Marty," I begged, "I appreciate your concern, but I must weigh my options." Pleadingly, I looked at the doctor for his response.

"There is only one alternative, but remember, my recommendation is still the same. I feel very strongly about you having surgery now rather than further delaying it. However, if you insist upon waiting, then you must at least have an MRI (magnetic resonance imaging; see the box and glossary), and the sooner the better."

"Fine," I said. "I'll go this week. Can you schedule it for me?"

"Check with the nurse on your way out and she'll take care of it for you." Silently, Marty and I left his office after arranging for the MRI. The earliest appointment we could obtain was three days away. Another wait.

ON THE morning of the MRI, I had initially wanted to drive downtown alone, but Mother and Dad insisted on accompanying me. Both in their eighties, they were so uptight about the simple test that Dad failed to pay attention to the road and nearly had a head-on collision. A real comedy ensued as I concentrated on calming them down.

Uterine and Ovarian Cancer

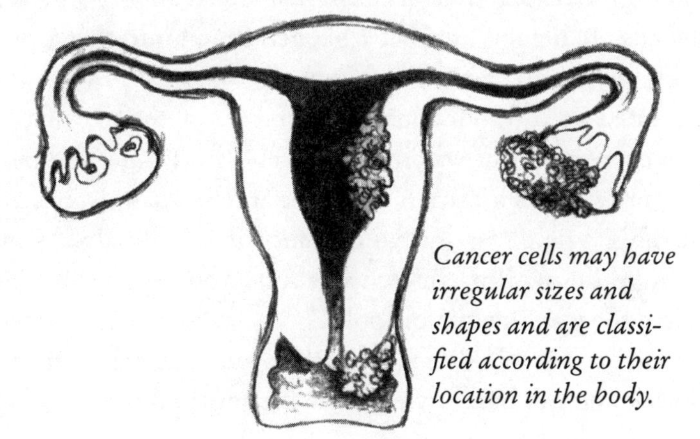

Cancer cells may have irregular sizes and shapes and are classified according to their location in the body.

For someone like me who has never experienced an MRI, the procedure can be both intimidating and claustrophobic. Lying flat on my back, I was wheeled into a tunnel and told not to move. I closed my eyes and tried to imagine myself anywhere other than inside that cavernous space. It was deathly quiet, almost like an out-of-body experience. Were it not for an occasional command from the technician, I might have felt completely detached from reality. After what seemed like an interminably long time (forty-five minutes in actuality), the ordeal was over. But was it? I was informed it would be another twenty-four hours before knowing the results of the pictures that had been taken. The doctor phoned with the results the next evening.

"Do you want the good news first or the bad news, Nancy?" he asked.

"I'll take the good news, Doctor."

"The good news is that you definitely have a large fibroid. The further good news is that the ovaries are not involved."

"Well, that's great, Doctor! So what's the bad news?"

"The bad news is that I think the tumor is malignant."

"But, Doctor, wait a minute. I've been doing my homework and am under the impression that 98 percent of all fibroids are benign. Isn't that true?"

"Actually the percentage is even higher than that."

"I don't understand! You're telling me that about 99 percent of all fibroids are benign but that *I* happen to fall into that 1 percent category that's malignant. Why?"

"Because your tumor apparently grew from the size of a pea to the size of a grapefruit within a relatively short time, and because you go for regular six-month checkups and this has just been diagnosed. This type of fast-growing tumor is usually always malignant. In addition, I'm concerned about your symptoms, and I don't like the way this tumor looks."

"Then do you think it might be the prudent thing for me to call my doctor and ask him just when he first noticed this condition?"

"Absolutely."

Immediately I dialed Dr. Kass's office. Within moments Dr. Kass was on the line. He quickly put my mind at ease by informing me that he had been tracking my condition for about three and a half years but hadn't wanted to alarm me. Most women, he said, develop small polyps and sometimes even fibroids. Although he had informed me some time ago of the presence of these polyps, it was of no great concern because I knew it was common to many women. Moreover, polyps tend to disappear over time without treatment.

Years ago it was common practice to perform hysterectomies on women for any abnormality such as polyps or small fibroids. However, this practice has become less popular over the last ten years, and today hysterectomies should only be performed as a last resort. The guideline now used by most physicians is to recommend surgery when a woman's enlarged uterus with fibroid growth is bigger than a twelve-week pregnancy. Of course, there's a trade-off. If a fibroid is removed while it's still small, then a vaginal hysterectomy can easily be performed. This procedure involves a shorter recovery period with far less pain and no visible scar. But, because many of these fibroids disappear naturally, it is better to avoid such drastic and costly measures whenever possible. Therefore, the more conservative approach is to wait and see.

When it appears that the fibroid is becoming too large, an abdominal hysterectomy is then unavoidable. This occurs most frequently in women who enter menopause after age fifty.

Drug therapy is sometimes used for relief of symptoms associated with abnormal bleeding and chronic pelvic pain as well as fibroid tumors. It has been proven that drug therapy for abnormal bleeding and chronic pelvic pain can produce significant reductions in symptoms after three months and is sustained after twelve months. Because a woman's natural supply of estrogen is responsible for causing these conditions, a hormone-blocking drug is used to counteract the problem. However, a drug therapy program produces *pseudo-menopause* until the drugs are stopped. Pretreatment symptoms often reappear at the completion of therapy. Women treated nonsurgically for fibroids have reported even fewer successes with drug therapy even though the drugs were temporarily effective in shrinking the tumors.[6]

> *Years ago it was common practice to perform hysterectomies on women for any abnormality such as polyps or small fibroids. However, this practice has become less popular over the last ten years, and today hysterectomies should only be performed as a last resort.*

Breakthrough bleeding, or spotting, between menstrual flows is usually harmless, although it could also be a signal that something is wrong. Uterine cancer, endometrial polyps, hyperplasia, and fibroid tumors are among the conditions that require medical attention. After evaluating your condition, your doctor may recommend a dilatation and curettage (D&C) and/or surgery. On the other hand, it could be a condition that is treatable with medication or a change of hormones.

Abnormally heavy bleeding must never be ignored. If this occurs, phone your doctor. Postmenopausal women sometimes have brief episodes of vaginal bleeding even though their normal menstrual cycle has ceased. Only when other symptoms occur simultaneously and/or bleeding has resumed six months or more after the menstrual cycle has stopped can it be assumed there may be a problem.

My initial reaction regarding surgery was fear—fear of being unconscious, fear of loss, fear of pain, fear of death. Fear can be paralyzing, or it can be energizing. Most people who are paralyzed by fear can "move" to a place where fear can be used as an energizer. This movement is accomplished by allowing yourself to look at your fears. What specifically are you afraid of? Make a list of your specific fears—for example, the fears of being unconscious, of suffering loss, of experiencing pain and even death. Very reasonable fears, wouldn't you say? Now ask yourself, What is it about those fears that make them so scary? The bottom line for most people is "control." Your fear is about being out of control. However, there are still things you can control. What are they? Get to work on those things you *can* control. Use the energy provided by your fear to get things accomplished. Fear can be the motivating force to seek answers and establish the truth about your condition. This is something you can control.

Although my fear initially robbed me of sleep and a normal appetite, it was my fear that also helped me evaluate a life-threatening situation. Rather than allowing myself to wallow in anxiety, a formidable obstacle, fear helped set me into action. My concerns about my upcoming surgery, fueled by my fears, afforded me a rare opportunity. Instead of thinking about the surgery with dread, I thought about it as a challenge. I could survive—and thrive!

AFTER SPEAKING with Dr. Kass, I felt I had been given a new lease on life. He had been my gynecologist for nearly ten years, and I had complete confidence in his professional judgment. Moreover, it is usually customary for a patient to return to his or her own doctor after consulting with another physician for a second opinion. Dr. Kass reassured me that it was almost certainly a benign fibroid and that waiting another three months for surgery would not endanger my life. I would be monitored every three weeks, and if the condition became too uncomfortable, we would then reevaluate the date of surgery. As of now, however, surgery was scheduled for the beginning of September.

Not until much later did I realize that the opinion of a second doctor not only might be more aggressive than the original physician's but that a specialist would look on the situation from his or her perspective and, in this case, that perspective was cancer. Had my condition been malignant, a cancer arising from muscle or fibrous tissue in the wall of the uterus is known as a *uterine sarcoma*. Sarcomas, if not caught in time, can be fatal.[7]

Even though I had further questions regarding the surgery, the most important one had been answered—the question of *survival.* My needing the hysterectomy was no longer disputed, but I had time to think. I could use this time to educate myself and more thoughtfully formulate my medical questions. What I discovered was that the greatest fear of all is fear of the unknown, but the most powerful force is—the will to survive.

CHAPTER TWO

FIBROIDS *and* ENDOMETRIOSIS

BEFORE WE continue, let's take a closer look at two conditions many women face that threaten their physical health. The next two chapters highlight the importance of self-empowerment through acquisition of information, which increases your sense of control and thereby abates your fear. This chapter, then, aims to help you do just that.

Fibroids and endometriosis are similar conditions in that they entail material growing unnaturally in or around a woman's uterus; both can be quite painful. They differ, though, in terms of treatment. Some type of hysterectomy is often necessary for a woman with fibroids; in fact, fibroids are the most common reason for a hysterectomy. Endometriosis, on the other hand, is less common and can usually be treated more conservatively. Sometimes it is not until the surgeon is operating to remove fibroids that endometriosis is also discovered.

FIBROIDS

In a well-written handbook titled *Uterine Fibroids: What Every Woman Needs to Know,* the author, Nelson Stringer, M.D., educates women about different surgical alternatives to hysterectomy. He also thoroughly describes the surgical techniques used by highly skilled surgeons. Some of the information that follows is taken from that book.[1]

Estimates are that about one-fifth to one-fourth of adult females develop fibroid tumors, but these estimates are believed to be low because not all women with fibroids have symptoms. Moreover, the incidence of fibroid tumors is higher in African-American women. One study showed that 45 percent of African-American women between the ages of thirty and thirty-nine had fibroid tumors. Another study indicated that 45 percent of Caucasian women and 58 percent of African-American women had hysterectomies for fibroids. (Keep in mind, though, that this study was conducted in 1989 when the tendency to perform hysterectomies was greater than it is today.) The point of these studies is that many women have fibroids, yet not all require hysterectomies. Additionally, there are alternatives to hysterectomy.

Fibroids develop out of the lining of the uterus, which is really a muscle (the uterine muscles' contractions are what cause cramps). Although a fibroid begins its growth in the lining of the uterus, it may not remain there. Sometimes it will develop a "stalk" from which the fibroid hangs. If the stalk grows to the outside of the uterus, it is known as a *subserosal fibroid* and is very easy to remove (a hysterectomy is not required). If the stalk of the fibroid grows toward the inside of the uterus so that the fibroid "hangs" inward from the lining of the uterus, it is known as a *submucosal fibroid*. Sometimes this type of fibroid protrudes from the opening of the cervix into the vagina. No matter where these inward-growing submucosal fibroids occur, they usually cause heavy menstrual flow. A third type, the *intramural fibroid*, remains within the lining of the uterus and grows there. These fibroids, along with the subserosal type, are the most common.

Fibroid sizes are usually compared to the size of a pregnant uterus or (believe it or not) fruits. For a point of reference, consider that a normal uterus is equivalent to the size of a small pear. The size of the uterus right before childbirth is about the size of a watermelon. Fibroid sizes vary from small to large: orange, grapefruit, melon, pineapple, pumpkin.

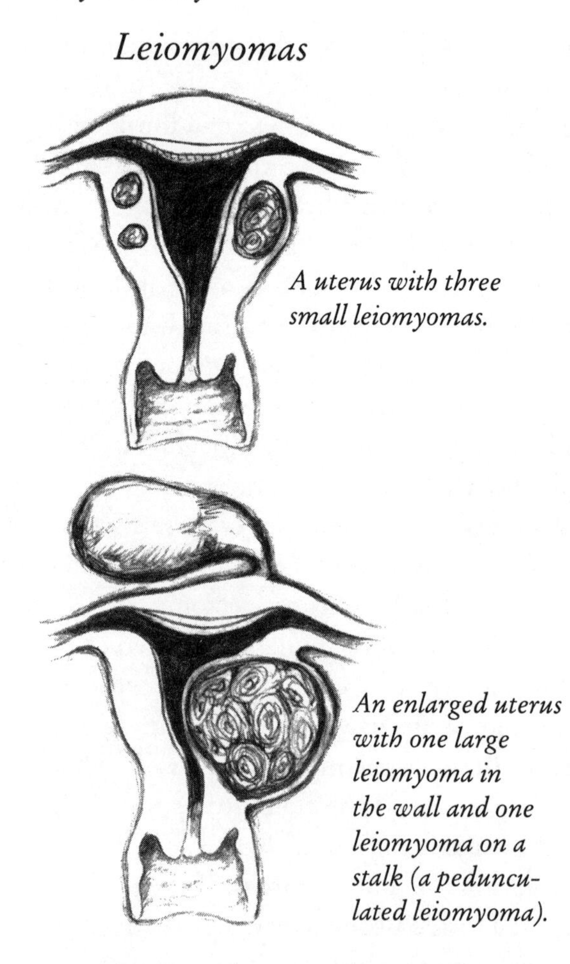

Leiomyomas

A uterus with three small leiomyomas.

An enlarged uterus with one large leiomyoma in the wall and one leiomyoma on a stalk (a pedunculated leiomyoma).

Symptoms of fibroids include heavy menstrual bleeding, pelvic pain, pelvic pressure, sudden urge to urinate, stress incontinence (unintentional loss of urine during coughing or lifting), and rectal pressure.

Factors Affecting Fibroid Growth

Although much remains to be learned about what causes fibroids, we do know that fibroids are estrogen-dependent. In other words, the more estrogen you have circulating in your bloodstream, the more likely you are to develop fibroids. Lifestyle factors that affect the amount of circulating estrogen will thus also affect the likelihood of developing fibroids. Body fat is a major source of estrogen. Therefore, if you have a high percentage of body fat, you are at increased risk to develop fibroids.

You do not have to look fat to have a higher-than-average percentage of body fat; women with underdeveloped muscles tend to have a higher percentage of body fat. (An average level of body fat for a woman is about 25 percent.) Regular exercise, including some modest (not bodybuilding) weight lifting, will help reduce your percentage of body fat. Swimming is not particularly helpful in reducing body fat levels because regular swimmers' bodies naturally develop a protective layer of fat under their skin to help keep them warm in the water.

Symptoms of fibroids include heavy menstrual bleeding, pelvic pain, pelvic pressure, sudden urge to urinate, stress incontinence (unintentional loss of urine during coughing or lifting), and rectal pressure.

Other factors influence the development of fibroids; most seem to be in some way related to the production of estrogen. For example, the more full-term pregnancies you have had, the less likely you are to develop fibroids. Similarly, if you have been on oral contraceptives for at least ten years, the likelihood of developing fibroids is reduced by about 30 percent. But take heed! Once a fibroid starts to grow, the extra estrogen in oral contraceptives causes fibroids to grow more rapidly. Cigarette smoking decreases the risk of fibroids, although this is no reason not to quit. Also, postmenopausal women have a decreased incidence of fibroids.

Once a fibroid starts to grow, its rate of growth depends on the number of estrogen receptors the fibroid has and the amount of estrogen circulating in the body. Decreasing levels of estrogen result in decreasing rates of growth. However, no known dietary changes or herbal remedies will cause a fibroid to shrink. If you already have fibroids, your best nonsurgical option may be to attempt to reduce the rate of growth through a low-fat diet and exercise until other nonsurgical options become available or you pass through menopause (when fibroids naturally shrink). The only other natural way that fibroids shrink is during pregnancy. Fibroids diminish in size during pregnancy either because levels of progesterone (which neutralizes the effects of estrogen) increase or because the growing fetus lowers the blood supply to the fibroid. Dying fibroids may cause severe pain during pregnancy and are managed with pain medications and bed rest.

Treating Fibroids

Conservative management of the symptoms of fibroids includes anti-inflammatory drugs such as ibuprofen and hormone-based drugs (synthetic gonadotropin-releasing hormones) that shrink fibroids. Gonadotropin-releasing hormones (GnRH) are typically used before surgery to shrink the fibroid to a more manageable size before the fibroid is removed. Once GnRH drugs are stopped, the fibroid will begin to return to its larger size, so these drugs are just a temporary intervention. Side effects from GnRH drugs are most often in the form of hot flashes; 85 percent of women experience hot flashes as a result of taking GnRH drugs.

The size of the fibroid, the type (intramural, subserosal, submucosal), and its location in relation to the blood supply determine the type of procedure that can be used to treat the fibroid. In some cases, medication can be used to shrink it. In other cases, the artery that provides the blood supply to the fibroid is blocked using a procedure called *arterial embolization*. In this procedure the surgeon inserts a catheter into an artery in the woman's leg and moves the catheter within the artery up to where the artery supplies the fibroid. At this supply point a foam (Gelfoam) or plastic (propylvinyl alcohol) is injected into the artery to block the blood flow. Pelvic pain follows and may last up to twelve hours after the procedure. Fibroids shrink over a period of months to as much as 80 percent or as little as 20 percent of the original size. This procedure is not recommended for women who desire to become pregnant because it results in limited blood supply to the uterus.

Six surgical options are also available for removing a fibroid. Three types of total hysterectomy comprise half of these options. These three types—a total (transabdominal) hysterectomy, a vaginal hysterectomy, and a laparoscopic-assisted vaginal hysterectomy (LAVH)—each result in the loss of the uterus, fallopian tubes, and, consequently, periods. The financial cost for these procedures is approximately the same, and the time before you can return to everyday activities, including sex, is estimated to be six to seven weeks.

The difference between these three alternatives is in the process of removing your internal organs and, as a result, the length of your hospital stay. In the *total transabdominal hysterectomy,* an incision is made in your abdomen, and the uterus and fallopian tubes are removed through the incision. The surgeon need not have specialized skills to perform this type of surgery. The length of stay in the hospital is three to five days. In a *vaginal hysterectomy* and *LAVH,* the organs are removed through the vagina, which reduces the hospital stay to one to two days. The differences between the vaginal hysterectomy and the LAVH are the location and type of incision. The LAVH uses a laparoscope to make small incisions in the abdomen and to disconnect the organs before removal through the vagina, whereas a vaginal hysterectomy makes an incision in the vagina.

The other three nonhysterectomy options for removing fibroids are open myomectomy, laparoscopic myomectomy, and hysteroscopic myomectomy. The word *myomectomy* means that your internal organs remain intact. An *open myomectomy* has a similar recovery time to the total hysterectomy, probably because both procedures entail a relatively large incision in the abdomen. According to Dr. Stringer, 99 percent of fibroids can be removed through an open myomectomy (without the loss of your internal organs), but many physicians hesitate to offer this alternative because it is a more difficult surgical procedure with a greater likelihood of excessive bleeding (so you must donate your blood before the surgery). If your physician did not offer this surgical procedure as an option, it is wise to seek a second opinion. Doctors who are not comfortable with or knowledgeable about this operation will likely not mention it.

Additionally, in 1996 the cost for an open myomectomy was about $2,000 more than that for a total hysterectomy. Because of this increased expense, your health insurance may not cover it.

This is also an important point to discuss with your doctor, because some physicians may feel constrained to perform only "covered" surgical procedures.

The two other surgical options available for the removal of fibroids can sometimes be performed on an outpatient basis: the laparoscopic myomectomy and the hysteroscopic myomectomy. The difference between these two procedures is the way the fibroid is removed. *Laparoscopic myomectomy* is a high-tech surgery that uses specialized surgical instruments (tiny cameras, lasers, and electrosurgical instruments) to cut away the fibroid after the abdomen has been distended with carbon dioxide gas. This technique requires a very experienced laparoscopic surgeon. As a result, the cost is about $2,000 more than a total hysterectomy (in 1996), so be sure to check your medical insurance coverage. The good news is that a laparoscopic myomectomy appears to be suitable for most fibroids. Your expected hospital stay is one day, and your time until returning to everyday activities is one week.

If you have submucosal fibroid (the kind that hangs from a stalk toward the inside of your uterus), a *hysteroscopic myomectomy* can be performed. This procedure uses water to fill and distend the uterus. Using the hysteroscope (which includes lights and camera), the surgeon shaves the fibroid from the inside of the uterus. This procedure can usually be performed on an outpatient basis. The cost is about one-third of a total hysterectomy, and you can return to normal activities in about three days.

Future treatment of fibroids includes the use of the abortion pill RU-486 to shrink fibroids for the long term. This drug treatment has received preliminary approval for use in the nonsurgical management of fibroids by the Food and Drug Administration as of 1996.

ENDOMETRIOSIS

Endometriosis is an extremely painful disease that affects 10 to 20 percent of women between the ages of twenty and forty. In this condition, material is found outside the uterus that ordinarily lines the uterine walls and gets flushed out each month at the end of a woman's monthly cycle. When the uterine lining grows outside the womb as well as inside, it causes internal bleeding each month and painful menstrual periods. For women in their childbearing years, this condition can cause or worsen infertility problems. Symptoms include pain before and during your menstrual period, pain during intercourse, and infertility. A helpful book, *What Women Can Do About Chronic Endometriosis* by Judith Sachs, provided some of the information that follows.[2]

Factors Affecting Endometriosis

Doctors don't know how or why endometriosis occurs, and it is not something that is easily detected. Although the cause remains unknown, many theories and myths attempt to explain endometriosis. The *retrograde menstruation theory,* which is the most

Examples of Endometriosis

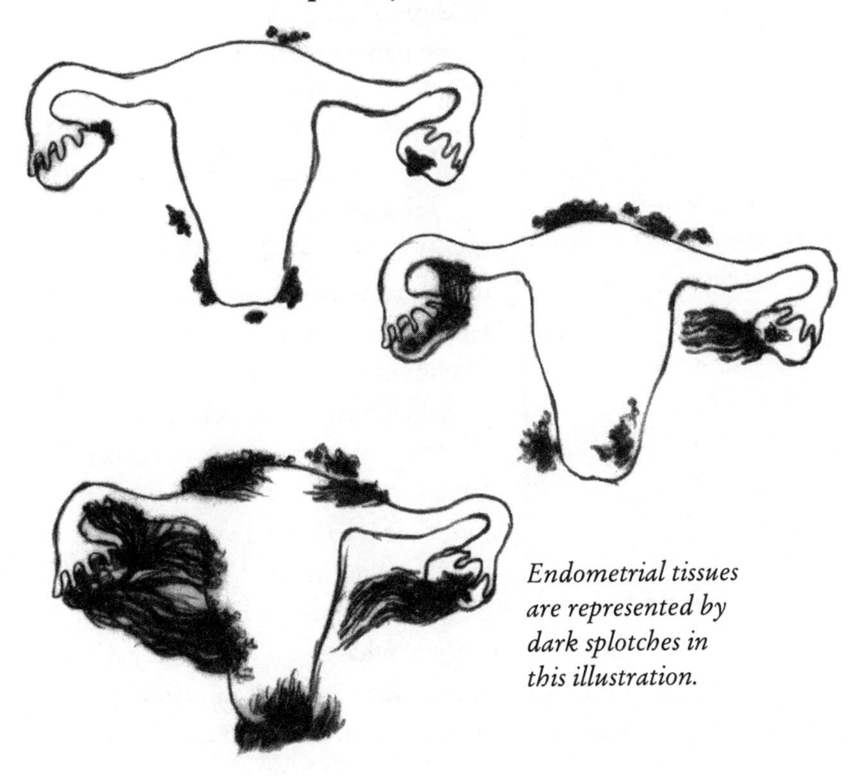

Endometrial tissues are represented by dark splotches in this illustration.

commonly accepted explanation of endometriosis, states that the menstruation flow fails to leave the body completely during menstruation but instead "backs up" in the fallopian tubes, all the way up to the ovaries and perhaps out past the ovaries into the pelvic cavity. Although it is true that 90 percent of women have this retrograde menstruation, not all of these women have endometriosis. This theory fails to account for the women who have retrograde menstruation but do not develop endometriosis.

The *autoimmune deficiency theory* states that because all women with retrograde menstruation do not get endometriosis, the women who do develop it are those with a weakened immune system. As the theory goes, women with strong immune systems are able to absorb the "backed-up" material when it enters the pelvic cavity, whereas women with weak autoimmune systems cannot. Some support for this theory comes from data showing that women with endometriosis usually suffer from other medical conditions related to autoimmune deficiency such as psoriasis, colitis, or yeast infections. If this theory is correct, a healthy lifestyle can help boost a weakened autoimmune system.

Misconceptions about endometriosis include the belief that it is limited to unmarried career women, that it results from tampon use, that it results from sexual intercourse during menstruation, and that a hysterectomy will eliminate endometriosis.

Another theory is the *iatrogenic theory*. *Iatrogenic* means that the condition has been caused by a medical intervention. Suspected iatrogenic causes of endometriosis are invasive diagnostic procedures, such as laparoscopy or biopsy, during the menstrual period, which may cause the menstrual blood to escape into the pelvic cavity and attach to other internal sites. In addition to endometriosis, other illness may be iatrogenic. For example, many women have developed a yeast infection after taking antibiotics; in this case, the yeast infection is iatrogenic in origin. Therefore, it is important to undertake any type of medical intervention with prudence, because you may experience unexpected consequences.

Misconceptions about endometriosis include the belief that it is limited to unmarried career women, that it results from tampon use, that it results from sexual intercourse during menstruation, and that a hysterectomy will eliminate endometriosis. Hysterectomy has not been shown to be an effective treatment for endometriosis in every case, because some women who have had a hysterectomy continue to suffer from endometriosis.

Treating Endometriosis

Conservative, nonsurgical treatment of endometriosis should be pursued whenever feasible. Dietary changes and herbal supplements are probably only effective in the very early stages of the disease, if at all. Physicians frequently prescribe the drug Danazol, a synthetic form of the male hormone testosterone, for mild to moderate endometriosis. It disrupts a woman's normal hormone cycle, monthly periods cease, and endometriosis diminishes as a result. However, while taking Danazol, many women experience masculinizing side effects, including increased muscle size, decreased breast size, and lowered voice. Other possible side effects are acne, hot flashes, nausea, headache, increased LDLs (low-density lipoproteins, or "bad" cholesterol), and liver dysfunction. The duration of treatment with Danazol is usually limited and dependent on the severity of the side effects. When the treatment is stopped, endometriosis may return.

Several new drugs have received preliminary approval by the FDA for the treatment and prevention of endometriosis. Preliminary use of the drug aromatase inhibitor has been shown to result in the rapid decrease in pelvic pain and almost complete elimination of endometriosis. RU-486 has also been shown effective in treating endometriosis in clinical studies.

A good source of up-to-date information about endometriosis is the Endometriosis Research Center, a nonprofit education and treatment organization. It can be found on the Internet at *www.endocenter.org/*.

CHAPTER THREE

"BUT I DON'T WANT *a* HYSTERECTOMY"

USUALLY WHEN your doctor first suggests that a hysterectomy may be necessary, disbelief quickly follows. You have been surprised to discover that you cannot remember what was said after the word *hysterectomy* was uttered. The remainder of that office visit is forever a blank. This "blanking-out" response is your mind's reaction to the idea that you may be in serious physical danger (either because you will be undergoing major surgery or because the fact that you need a hysterectomy signals that a condition is threatening your life). After leaving the doctor's office, you may have a feeling of unreality, like this cannot possibly be true. There must be some mistake. This disbelief response is the result of your mind struggling to accept and assimilate information that doesn't fit with what you have been thinking. You can use this response to activate your search for additional information, discover treatment alternatives, and formulate questions to be asked at a future date. Additionally, you may feel afraid or overwhelmed. Having these feelings means that the reality of what you are up against is sinking in; your mind is beginning to accept the new information and is "trying on" different scenarios, different outcomes. You may not yet have begun to consider your resources.

Realize that the disbelief and blanking out responses, fear, and feeling overwhelmed are normal and transient. They are not permanent states of mind, but while they are in control they get in the way of your thinking things through. The goal is to move yourself out of your automatic responses into a state that is more adaptive for you, a state in which you are ready to gather information and think about your alternatives in a calm, intelligent way. First, it is important to get yourself to realize that nothing has happened yet. You are the same person you were before you entered the doctor's office. You have a challenge ahead, but you have faced challenges in the past and can do it again. You really are still in control of the situation. You have choices. A hysterectomy cannot be performed without your permission. You may have alternatives.

RESPONSES TO REALITY

Once the idea that you may have to undergo a hysterectomy becomes more real to you, you may feel angry. "Why me?" you say and "Why now?" Depending on your personality, your anger may cause you to feel like a victim, avoid taking responsibility, close down and withdraw, become irritable and impatient, do something impulsive, wallow in resentment, or become pessimistic or defiant. Good ways to counteract your anger are with positive action. Some alternatives to anger are (1) using positive self-talk (e.g., "I can beat this"); (2) putting things into perspective (e.g., "A hysterectomy is not the worst thing that could happen to me"); (3) becoming involved in the decision making by becoming more knowledgeable (begin information gathering); (4) maintaining your sense of humor (make an effort to enjoy every moment of your life); and (5) engaging in activities that relax you (exercise, deep breathing, positive visualizations). Let's take a closer look now specifically at information gathering, which also gets covered in a different way in the following chapter.

GATHERING INFORMATION

The information-gathering stage is a very important way to use your anger constructively. Although getting necessary information may not be as simple as checking in *Consumer Reports* magazine, the information is out there. Information provided here is to help educate you about alternatives to hysterectomy and get you started on your own research. Every woman's situation is unique; therefore, the information you will need is unique. This book's information is *not* intended to replace medical advice that you would receive from a qualified medical professional. It *is* intended to help you decide what to discuss with, and even *suggest* to, your doctor.

Alternative Medicine For some women alternative medicine is an option (see the box "Terms to Understand" and the glossary for descriptions of some forms of alternative medicine). Holistic medicine, for example, originated in China at the turn of the century and is now gaining widespread attention and acceptance in Western culture. This approach offers attractive new therapies that consider the total person, body and soul, rather than concentrating on specific symptoms. Patients are instructed to listen to their bodies and be responsible for their own health maintenance. Emphasis is on moderation—sensible eating habits, proper rest, and regular (not strenuous) exercise.

Remember: prudent information gathering means that you explore all your options—alternative and traditional. Sometimes a combination of treatments might work best for your unique condition and symptoms.

The Chinese concept of *yin* (female) and *yang* (male), two opposite but complementary energies, is the basis for this theory. *Qi*, body energy, flows from organ to organ as it supplies and revitalizes the system. "According to this theory, menopause is a kidney-yin deficiency. The kidney controls or encompasses the ovaries and uterus; we're missing yin, which is feminine."[1]

Remember: prudent information gathering means that you explore all your options—alternative and traditional. Sometimes a combination of treatments might work best for your unique condition and symptoms. Most important, a smart patient should not ignore the advice of her primary caregiver in favor of an alternative medical solution used exclusively.

If you are surprised at the idea that you may actually make suggestions to your doctor, then you are still thinking that your doctor has all the answers. That's just not true. Actually, a good doctor knows that he or she does not have all the answers. A good doctor also knows that the field of medicine is constantly evolving because of advances in technology, research, pharmaceuticals, and changes in thinking resulting from input from professionals in related fields, such as acupuncturists, herbalists, and homeopathic physicians. Because of this evolution, new information is obtained and techniques are developed almost on a daily basis. Although we try to provide comprehensive and balanced information about hysterectomy and alternative treatments, the information is constantly changing.

A Word About Experts Experts generally have a clear point of view and are very knowledgeable in an area of specialization. Generally, the more specialized the area, the narrower the point of view. The opposite holds true as well. The more general a person's knowledge base, the less he or she may know about any specific area. Also, the type of work an expert does biases that person's opinion toward a specific type of solution. For example, imagine you have had a headache for two weeks. You go to an ob/gyn and she checks your hormone levels; you go to a brain surgeon and he looks for brain tumors; you go to an acupuncturist and he does acupuncture; you go to a naturopath and she looks at your diet. You get the idea. Although this example is a little exaggerated, it is important to keep in mind that everyone, even an expert, is biased in some way. An expert feels most comfortable operating and making recommendations in his or her area of expertise. Therefore, talk to experts from many different orientations to get the best idea about your options and the most well-rounded view of your situation.

TERMS TO UNDERSTAND

Acupuncture—The practice of inserting fine needles into specific points on the body, this technique is supposed to help alleviate pain and symptoms while restoring the flow of bodily energy and balance.

Homeopathy—Homeopathy is a botanical alternative medicine based on the premise that a disease can be treated with small doses of the same substance that initially caused it. In the case of fibroids, for example, it has been reported that they tend to shrink and symptoms are alleviated when the correct homeopathic remedy is applied. Herbal treatment is also used for the relief of menopausal symptoms, such as hot flashes.

Magnetic therapy—This alternative treatment is one of the latest and most innovative forms of alternative medicine. The theory behind applying magnets for therapeutic use is that you are letting your body's natural

A Word About Scientific Research Although scientific research is the best we have in terms of objective information about what works and what doesn't, the conclusions made as a result of scientific research are not always correct. Usually false conclusions are due to an error that nobody noticed. The false conclusion is a result of the way the research was done. This type of error affects the generalizability of the conclusions. For example, it used to be that most medical research was done with men and was generalized to women. As a result, it was thought that alcohol affected both men and women alike, which is not true. Alcohol can interact with estrogen replacement therapy (ERT) and increase the level of estrogen in the blood. Obviously, this information could not have been obtained by studying men. It was not until recently that researchers realized that a woman's physiology is different from a man's and thus responds differently from a man's. Research outcomes in all-male studies, therefore, do not necessarily apply to women.

Sometimes the incorrect conclusion results from a bias that is so widely held that it is years before the bias is questioned. The healing capabilities alleviate pain and stress. When a magnet is applied to the body, the assumption is that magnetic waves pass through body tissue while stimulating blood flow to the circulatory system. Next, the lymphatic system takes over, carrying the toxins away from the body so the healing process can begin.

For more information about alternative medical procedures and where to get help in your area, contact: the National Women's Health Information Center at 1-800-994-WOMAN or

The American Holistic Medical Association
4101 Lake Boone Trail, Suite 201
Raleigh, NC 27607
(919) 787-5181

questioning of the bias comes from a change in thinking that occurs many years later, when the long held beliefs come into question. For example, in 1966 Robert A. Wilson, M.D., published the book *Feminine Forever* in which he characterized menopause as an estrogen deficiency disease, which if left untreated resulted in the loss of femininity. His assumption was that a postmenopausal woman could not retain her femininity without the use of drugs (i.e., ERT). By Dr. Wilson's definition, femininity is based on the physical appearance of a woman only. He gave no recognition to other attributes that typify femininity (and are not "treated" using ERT), such as the sound of her voice, her style of relating to others, what she values, the way she moves, how she expresses her feelings, and how she dresses and grooms herself. In other cultures that do not emphasize shallow physical attributes, menopause is considered an important passage that bestows increased wisdom, divine attributes, and prestige to a woman. It is the woman's inner self and not her physical appearance that is valued. In those cultures women have fewer negative symptoms such as osteoporosis, vaginitis, and hot flashes. Scientists and researchers have been unable to explain why the way the people in a culture think about menopause affects the symptoms of menopause. Perhaps it's a mind-body effect, in which thoughts affect physiology. Or perhaps there is no cause-effect relation at all between the cultural beliefs and menopausal symptoms, and the actual cause of the difference lies in the diets that these women of other cultures consume. This conundrum is an example of the "fuzziness" of science.

A SPECIAL COST-BENEFIT ANALYSIS

Once you have gathered information, you are prepared to enter the negotiation stage. This is not a negotiation with your doctor, although the doctor will be involved. A good doctor will listen to you and hear your concerns and consider your ideas. Your doctor will take the time to discuss matters with you and help you understand your options. The negotiation process referred to here has to do with the costs you are willing incur in relation to the potential benefits you expect to receive. These costs and benefits should be based not simply on what you imagine to be true but on a thorough search for accurate information.

> *A good doctor will listen to you and hear your concerns and consider your ideas.*

You must consider the consequences of going *without* a hysterectomy as well as the consequences of having one. The most common negative consequences of having a hysterectomy are the change in your ability to produce some or all of needed hormones, physical scarring, a period of physical and emotional healing, and the loss of ability to bear children. Positive outcomes include increased energy levels, elimination of symptoms, freedom from periods and pregnancy concerns, and riddance of a possible life-threatening medical condition.

You must take into consideration the condition(s) that made your doctor recommend the hysterectomy. Attempting to rid yourself of endometriosis is a different type of reason for pelvic surgery than attempting to survive a cancerous condition is. The first represents an attempt to end chronic pain and, as a result, improve the quality of your life. The second is about eliminating a condition that could kill you.

The decision may not only be whether to have pelvic surgery but what kind of surgery is appropriate for you, what type of pelvic surgery has been recommended, and what alternative, nonsurgical methods are available or being developed for your condition. You must consider the level of trust you have in the information you have acquired and how much you trust the experts to whom you have talked. Unfortunately, some unknowns will remain. However, it is certain that if you decide on a hysterectomy, the removal of your organs is final. They cannot be returned to you once they are removed.

With regard to the nature of the hysterectomy operation, perhaps more than one surgical procedure has been used for your condition (the various types of hysterectomies are described in Chapter 4). In that case, you may choose to acquire additional information, decide between alternatives, and select your doctor carefully, based in part on the skills that she or he possesses. However, thoroughly researching the options in this manner incurs a higher "front-end cost" in terms of time and effort. You may feel too overwhelmed to be able to make such an investment of energy to do all this work. Not everyone has the luxury of enough time or easy access to information or experts. You can only do the best you can under your unique circumstances.

Perhaps lifestyle changes have been shown to affect your condition, but the results of these changes may take longer to have an effect, have a less certain outcome, and require commitment and self-discipline on your part. For example, you may choose to wait for menopause to occur naturally, when the change in your hormone levels could significantly improve or even reverse your condition. Before you become menopausal, you may take vitamin, mineral, and/or herbal supplements to lessen the symptoms associated with your condition. You may choose acupuncture and/or relaxation training to help you manage your pain. You may start an exercise program and change your diet because those changes have been shown to slow down the worsening of your condition. Supplements, relaxation, diet, and exercise are not quick fixes; they are the building blocks of a healthy lifestyle.

Keep in mind, however, there is no guarantee that your condition will improve or when it will improve. Usually changes such as these have an effect over a period of months, not hours or days. Your personal tolerance for slow improvement in your condition, uncertainty regarding the final outcome, as well as your ability to initiate and maintain the changes you choose must be considered and evaluated realistically and in relation to your condition. Some women are so overburdened that they cannot find the time or energy to make these types of changes.

These decisions are difficult ones. A diagnosis of cancer has serious life-death ramifications, yet there are documented incidences of unexplained spontaneous remission. Conversely, it is unlikely that anyone ever died of endometriosis. However, the pain associated with some forms of endometriosis can be so unbearable that the sufferer may wish she were dead. A woman may become paralyzed with indecision and is relieved to do what the doctor suggests. Another, so overwhelmed by the inherent uncertainties, chooses to "get it over with" as quickly as possible, just to be rid of the anxiety. Each situation is unique. Every woman has limits, so if you've reached yours, just do the best you can under the circumstances.

CHAPTER FOUR

PREPARING MIND *and* BODY

THE TASK of preparing for my surgery now lay ahead, and I began by making a list of things to do:

1. Read up on everything concerning fibroid tumors and hysterectomies.
2. Get the house in order.
3. Maintain a healthy diet and regular exercise program.
4. Plan meals for several weeks; cook and freeze them.

Surgery no longer was something to fear; instead, I chose to view it as an interesting new challenge. For the next three months I would be very busy. My new project did not take the place of my normal routine; it simply added a new dimension.

I continued to work three days a week and on nonworking days swam at the health club and used the gym. Staying in shape and following good nutritional habits and proper diet were high on my list of priorities. I also consulted with Dr. Kass about taking extra vitamins prior to surgery in addition to my daily regimen of one multivitamin plus two calcium tablets and vitamin E. To those he added vitamins B and C (important vitamins for the immune system). On my next appointment I was then prepared with a full list of written questions for Dr. Kass:

Question 1: Length of time in surgery?

Answer: Approximately one and a half to two hours.

Question 2: If I need a blood transfusion, should I store some now to avoid diseases such as AIDS?

Answer: Blood transfusions are rarely needed for this type of surgery.

Question 3: Length of a hospital stay?

Answer: Between three and five days is the average length of a stay for abdominal surgery. Less time is required for vaginal hysterectomies.

Question 4: Will you leave the cervix intact as well as the ovaries? If both ovaries are not healthy, would you save at least one or a piece of one so I don't go into menopause?

Answer: Because you're monogamous and in a low-risk category of developing cervical cancer, the cervix can be saved. Although we could try to save the ovaries, it's unlikely because the weight of a large fibroid pulls on the fallopian tubes, often elongating them. When this happens, nothing is left to support the tubes and ovaries, because the uterus is out. Nevertheless, you'll be placed on estrogen while you're still in the hospital so you won't suffer the effects of menopause.

Question 5: What possible complications are there?

Answer: Usually none, unless the patient has serious health problems such as heart disease or diabetes. But some bleeding or infection could occur, and in rare instances something gets nicked that wasn't meant to be cut.

Question 6: What about pain? What do you use to control it?

Answer: You'll feel pain around the incision, and the abdominal area will feel bruised. Two drugs normally used for pain are Demerol and morphine, either of which the patient can control by using a hand device. It is administered directly through an intravenous tube.

Question 7: When can I return to normal foods?

Answer: A normal diet can usually be resumed after the first twenty-four hours.

Question 8: What about bladder and bowel problems after abdominal surgery?

Answer: A catheter, attached to the bladder, will be inserted during surgery and normally is removed on the second day. Bowel problems usually do exist after abdominal surgery, but a liquid diet for the first day or two normally corrects the problem.

Question 9: Will I have an IV (an intravenous tube)? Any other tubes?

Answer: An IV tube will be the only one still remaining after surgery. During surgery an air tube is also inserted down the patient's throat to help with breathing but is removed in the recovery room or prior to leaving the operating room.

Question 10: Can you guarantee a bikini incision rather than a vertical one?

Answer: Bikini incisions are used most frequently today. Only when complications arise, and definitely in the case of a carcinoma, is a vertical incision considered. Size and location of a tumor are also taken into account.

Question 11: What type of stitch (or staples) will be used?

Answer: Many doctors prefer staples today because most believe that this method is less painful, heals more quickly, and has less scarring. It also takes less time and is therefore more cost-effective. Some doctors still prefer stitches, the more conventional method.

Question 12: Can I use vitamin E on the incision to help it heal faster?

Answer: You may apply vitamin E immediately after surgery.

Question 13: Is it safe to take prescribed drugs, used regularly, on the day of surgery?

Answer: This question usually must be cleared also with the attending anesthesiologist. Some doctors prefer the patient not to take anything after midnight on the evening before surgery. Some will agree that prescribed drugs may be taken on the morning of surgery with very little water.

Question 14: What will fill up the space once the tumor and female organs have been removed?

Answer: Organs resume normal position after tumor removal, and empty space closes up.

Question 15: How long for full recovery?

Answer: Full recovery may take up to one year before a patient feels like her old self, but usually within three to four months the abdominal area is no longer painful and normal activity can be enjoyed.

Question 16: When can I return to work? Have sex? Exercise?

Answer: Usually a patient can return to work five to six weeks after surgery. Six weeks for sex and exercise.

Because I was now aware of my thickening belly and occasional pain and discomfort, comfortable clothing became an issue. Anything fitted was out. Warm-up suits became a staple because they're easy to wear and extremely comfortable. I purchased a few new outfits to give myself a lift while providing extra comfort, and I made sure they were something I'd enjoy wearing even after surgery. Shopping was fun, and I enjoyed teasing the sales woman.

"I'm looking for a chic new outfit," I'd say, "but something semimaternity."

"Oh," came the dubious response, "and when are you expecting?"

"I'm 'expecting' a tumor the beginning of September," I replied tongue-in-cheek. Dead silence. After a moment of quiet I assured her that it was a planned surgery, and then the clerk would become exceedingly helpful.

EMPOWERING YOURSELF THROUGH KNOWLEDGE

Now that I accepted surgery, my main objective was to educate myself thoroughly regarding my medical condition and upcoming operation. It was, after all, my body, and I felt I had some say in the matter. Moreover, fear of the unknown is much greater than knowing ahead of time what to expect.

Both public libraries and bookstores offer a wealth of material on the general subject of women's health as well as specific topics such as (1) medical problems leading to surgery, (2) hysterectomies and surgical options, and (3) what to expect before and after a hysterectomy.

What I discovered was a wide range of opinions, especially between female and male physicians. Woman doctors, for example, were particularly sensitive to the emotional aspects of hysterectomy. They typically addressed such questions as these: What was the aftermath of the procedure, and how would it affect a woman's mental health? What about her physical health? Would a woman feel less female following a hysterectomy? What about a woman's sexual drive after surgery? Would her ability to experience pleasure during intercourse be in any way diminished? These, and many others, are natural concerns for all women facing a hysterectomy.

Now that I accepted surgery, my main objective was to educate myself thoroughly regarding my medical condition and upcoming operation. It was, after all, my body, and I felt I had some say in the matter.

HYSTERECTOMY DEFINED

To begin your research, peruse a small medical dictionary to define important terms. Most basic of them all is *hysterectomy,* so let's take a look at that term in general now and then more specifically. A *hysterectomy,* the removal of the uterus, is any surgical procedure involving removal of all or part of a woman's reproductive system. Fibroid tumors are the most common reason for performing a hysterectomy (see Chapter 2). An *ovariectomy* (or *oophorectomy*), the surgical removal of the ovaries, is frequently referred to as "castration" because it is somewhat equivalent to the removal of a man's testicles and triggers "instant menopause." However, an ovariectomy neither causes impotence nor prevents the ovariectomized woman from achieving orgasm.

Symptoms experienced after an ovariectomy includes hot flashes and vaginal dryness, due to the sudden absence of estrogen. Some women also report a diminished sexual appetite following this procedure because the ovaries supply valuable hormones to a woman's body. Nevertheless, the majority of women do feel better following surgery because former pain and discomfort have been eliminated. The use of HRT not only helps replenish a woman's natural supply of hormones but also greatly reduces the physical dangers that can arise postsurgically. The two most common conditions that HRT helps prevent are osteoporosis (a loss in bony substances producing brittleness and softening of bones) and heart disease. Most important to keep in mind, however, is the overriding fact that ovarian cancer remains the deadliest gynecologic malignancy affecting women and carries with it a low five-year survival rate.[1]

A Woman's Reproductive Organs

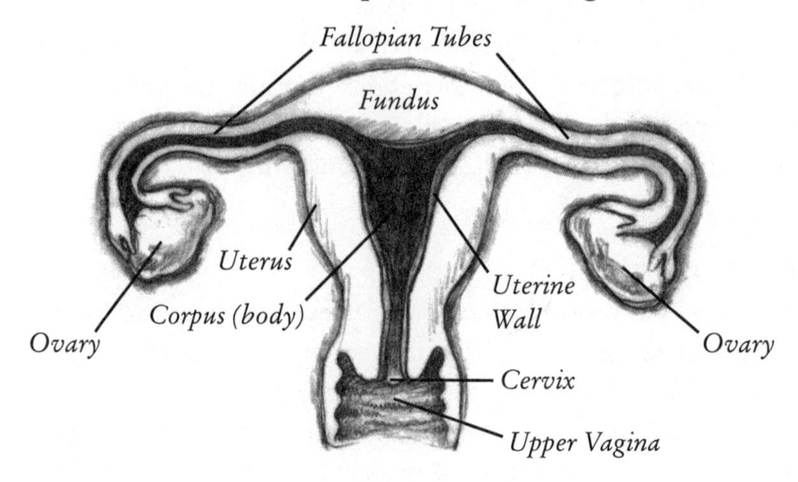

Several procedures are used today, most of which involve invasive surgery, but a vaginal hysterectomy still remains an option for some patients (see the box "Terms to Understand" and the glossary). With a *vaginal hysterectomy,* the uterus and cervix are removed but the fallopian tubes and ovaries remain intact.

The three most common types of invasive surgery include *subtotal hysterectomy, total hysterectomy,* and *total hysterectomy with bilateral salpingo-ovariectomy.*

A more recent technique is *laparoscopic surgery.* During a laparoscopic hysterectomy a tiny "Band-aid" incision is made at the belly button to insert the laparoscope (a lighted instrument, similar to a periscope). This procedure permits the doctor to look inside the body and examine the outside walls of the uterus and adjacent anatomical structures. Then several other small incisions are made to sever the uterine ligaments, blood vessels, and fallopian tubes. With this method scar tissue can be seen and cut out, cysts aspirated, ovaries removed, and even fibroids removed before the uterus is actually pushed out of the vagina.[2]

An Abdominal Hysterectomy

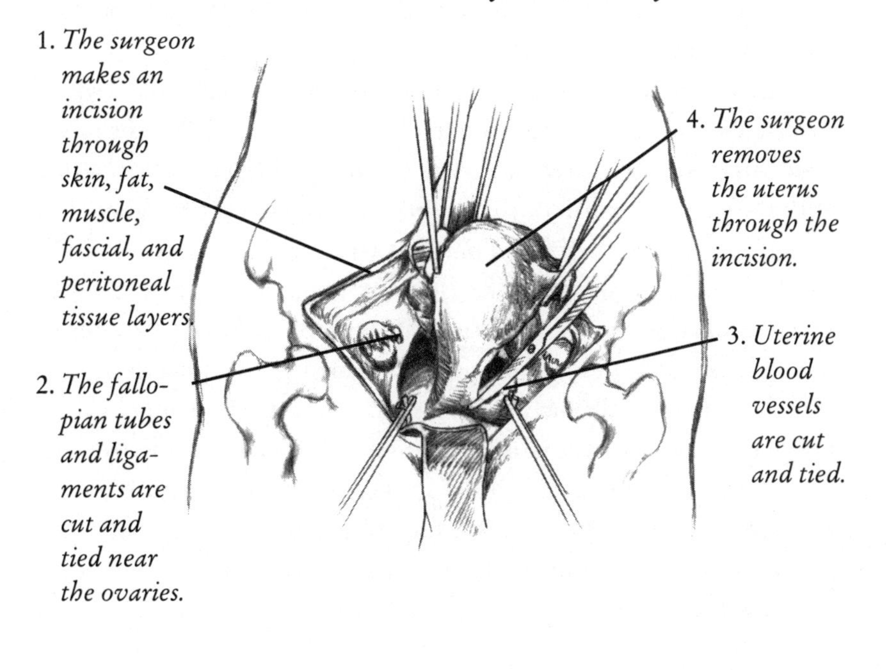

A Laparoscopic Vaginal Hysterectomy

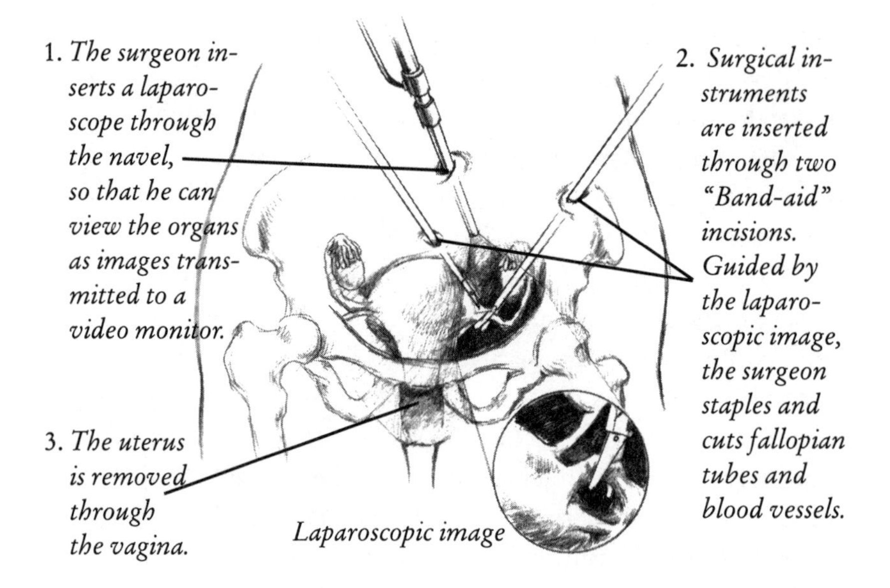

If your cervix is healthy, a single puncture in the navel can be used not only for the laparoscope but also for the uterus, fallopian tubes, and ovaries (if necessary). This is an alternative to the multiple incisions method and appropriate only if the cervix is healthy and to be retained.[3]

Seldom performed, and only in extreme cases, is the *radical hysterectomy*. This operation entails the removal of the entire reproductive system (uterus, cervix, ovaries, fallopian tubes) along with the upper portion of the vagina and affected lymph glands. It is usually performed only on patients with cervical cancer.

A final surgical option for some patients is myomectomy. A *myomectomy* removes *only* the diseased portion of the uterus, which is usually a fibroid or group of fibroids. Myomectomy was actually introduced nearly a century ago, yet it only gained popularity in recent years owing to modern medical technology. The operation is technically more complicated than a hysterectomy and definitely more time-consuming, taking up to four to six hours as opposed to one hour for an average hysterectomy. Not only is this procedure more expensive than a hysterectomy, but it does not

Types of Hysterectomies

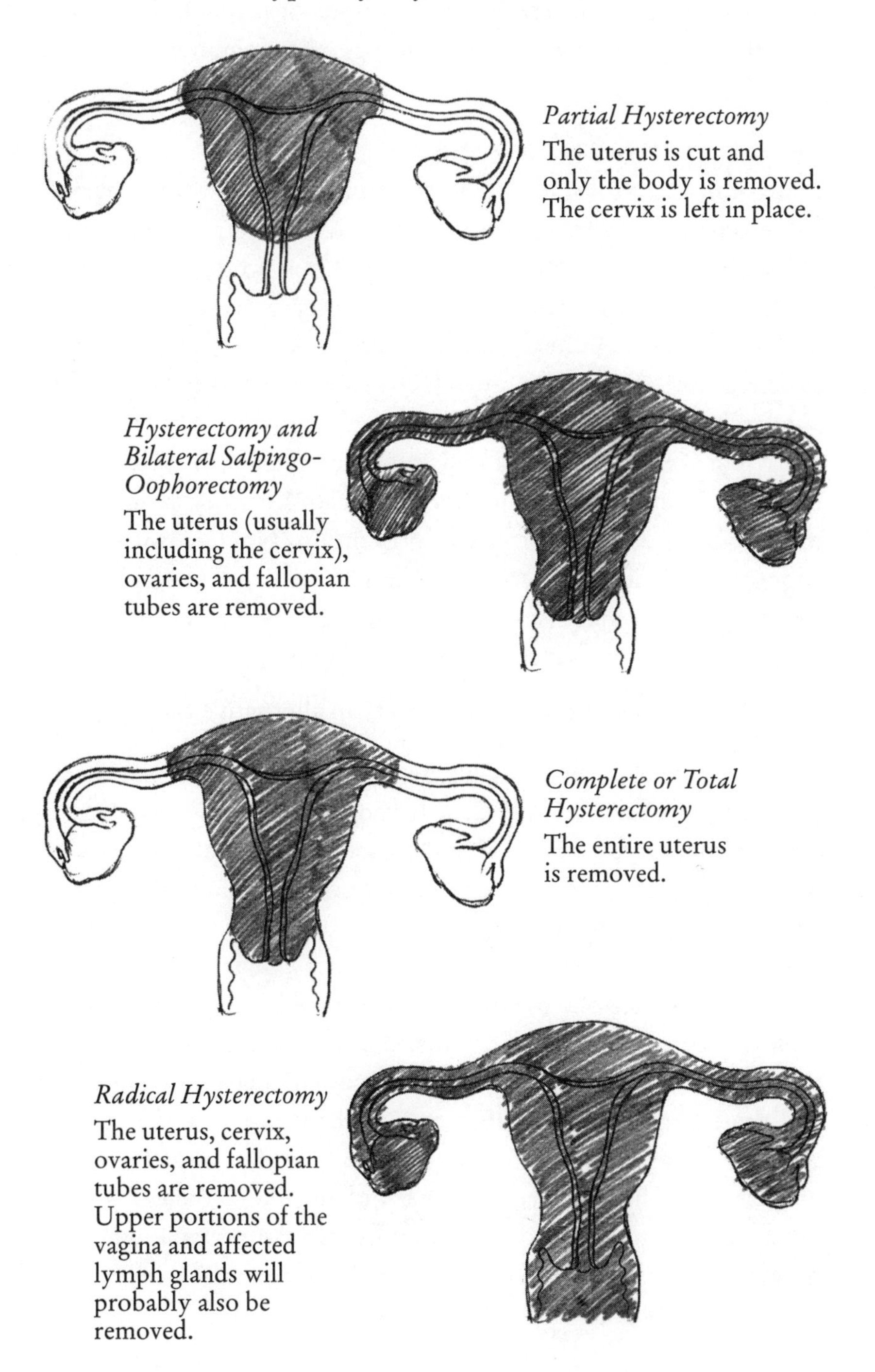

even guarantee that new fibroids won't develop postsurgically. This option, therefore, seems more impractical for most women with the exception of those still wanting to bear children.[4]

Other Points to Consider

Many considerations should be kept in mind for women facing hysterectomy. First, you must listen to your physician's advice before contemplating other options. There is no doubt that total hysterectomy with bilateral-salpingo ovariectomy is the most extensive approach because it eliminates all risk for a possible future cancer developing in the reproductive organs. Nevertheless, this approach is not for everybody.

A portion of the cervix still can be retained with this option even though it has been a matter of custom for forty years to remove it in its entirety for cancer prevention. Now, recent studies support new evidence that the cervix may actually have an important role in a woman's sexual response. Subsequent to these findings, some physicians strongly favor keeping the cervix because it is filled with nerve endings helpful to a woman's experiencing orgasm during intercourse.[5]

Some doctors also encourage their patients to keep their ovaries unless they are diseased. It had been common practice to remove the ovaries for all women past menopausal age because they were no longer felt to serve any purpose. That theory, however, is changing. Many of these same doctors now feel that ovaries not only play a significant part during coitus, but it is known that the ovaries (even old ovaries) provide valuable hormones for a woman's general well-being. Most commonly feared by women who want to keep their ovaries at all cost is that removing them and the estrogen they produce may lead to osteoporosis, cardiovascular disease, blood clotting, and the acceleration of the aging process. HRT helps prevent these problems. Nevertheless, it cannot be overemphasized that ovarian cancer can be fatal, which is why many physicians still favor removal of the ovaries when a hysterectomy is indicated.

TERMS TO UNDERSTAND

Laparoscopic vaginal hysterectomy—Removal of the uterus and possibly the cervix, ovaries, and fallopian tubes.

Myomectomy—Removal only of diseased portion of uterus, usually a fibroid or group of fibroids; more common for women who are still in their childbearing years and want to become pregnant.

Radical hysterectomy—Removal of the entire reproductive system, including a portion of the vagina.

Subtotal hysterectomy—Removal of the uterus but ovaries, fallopian tubes, and cervix are left in place.

Total hysterectomy—Removal of the uterus and cervix but not the ovaries or fallopian tubes.

Total hysterectomy with bilateral salpingo-ovariectomy—Removal of the uterus and cervix as well as the ovaries and fallopian tubes.

Vaginal hysterectomy—Removal of the uterus and cervix with the fallopian tubes and ovaries remaining intact.

With uterine tumors, the weight of the tumor often causes a prolapsed uterus, more commonly known as a tipped or fallen uterus. When this happens, the fallopian tubes become elongated, which usually necessitates the removal of the tubes and attached ovaries. Sometimes the uterus becomes weak and sags, a common condition for women who have had multiple pregnancies and haven't exercised their pelvic muscles.

In the final analysis, only those women with life-threatening problems or those whose symptoms severely affect the quality of their lives should submit themselves to surgery. Remember that your surgery may be optional, but reversing the surgery is not. Your doctor may have advised surgery as a remedy for your symptoms, but the aftermath of pelvic surgery will not be problem free.

In addition to its uncertain outcome, a hysterectomy is painful, both physically and sometimes emotionally. It is also expensive and irreversible. With the resultant permanent alterations you will have to alter your lifestyle slightly (e.g., the addition of HRT, regular exercise, perhaps a change in diet).

If you had hoped to avoid making lifestyle changes by having a hysterectomy, think again. Lifestyle changes are virtually unavoidable; they are a consequence of healthy aging. On the other hand, if surgery is the only viable option, then a positive approach toward the experience will have favorable results. In all aspects of life we have choices to make, and in dealing with choices there are trade-offs, both positive and negative. Doing nothing is also an option, and doing nothing has its consequences, too.

THROUGHOUT THE summer my life remained fairly normal, with just one exception—rearranging my life in preparation for the upcoming surgery. That proved beneficial because it all but eliminated a serious case of nerves and helped me focus on something other than the inevitable September date. Everyone's priorities are different; some will use their presurgery time to focus on their children, others will prepare for time away from their job, but for me it was a time to get my house in order.

Room by room, I began cleaning house as if I were doing a thorough spring cleaning. Closets and dresser drawers were emptied, rearranged, and unused items tossed or piled up for the Salvation Army. Then the carpeting was shampooed, furniture cleaned, house repairs made, and both air conditioning and heating systems were given their annual routine inspection. Nothing was overlooked so that the house, postsurgically, would be maintenance-free. Might this have been symbolic of a "new life"? Time to throw out the old to make room for the new?

> *In all aspects of life we have choices to make, and in dealing with choices there are trade-offs, both positive and negative.*

As a lover of nature and wildlife, I took this opportunity to improve the grounds around our home and extend our already existing wild bird sanctuary. Not only would bird-watching afford me hours of enjoyment during my recuperation, but it was also a healthy pastime, both physically and mentally—so much so that it became a passion. The more inclement the weather, the bigger the challenge and thus the greater my overall enjoyment.

Perhaps my most important task was planning and preparing meals, to be stored for after surgery. This task gave me peace of mind. Although I don't love cooking, it was an excellent way to consume hours of creative energy. If you are a list maker like I am, try writing down all your favorite dinner recipes. Next make the grocery lists and do the actual cooking, which does not need to be an onerous task. Just doubling the amount of food prepared each night for dinner and freezing half of it might be all that's necessary.

Pots of soup and applesauce, for example, are easy to portion into small containers for later use. All food can be clearly labeled and stored according to meat dishes, side dishes, and so forth. Even bread and pastries are freezable, and don't forget to store up on frozen vegetables. You may take shortcuts by adding prepared frozen foods such as TV dinners, pizzas, and casseroles serving four or more persons. Before you know it, you may have a freezer filled with plenty of food, literally from soup to nuts, to last several weeks. Best of all, you'll be completely self-sufficient in the kitchen department so you won't need to impose on well-meaning friends and relatives or order out. Eating fast food and carry-out from restaurants becomes not only monotonous but also very expensive.

While busying yourself with all these preparations, remember to reserve quality time for family and friends. We planned a family vacation for a few days that included our two adult sons, one's wife, and one's significant other.

At the same time we installed a new home computer, which sparked additional motivation to get on with the surgery and put it behind me so I could enjoy the new technology. Being finally connected to the World Wide Web, I'd be able to communicate globally on-line. The idea is to provide something interesting to occupy your time that will give you sufficient space for postsurgical recuperation. The computer was *my* method. What would work for you?

A FEW days before entering the hospital, I had my final preoperative visit with Dr. Kass. Everything seemed OK; the tumor didn't appear appreciably larger. Again, I stressed my concern over the type of incision and told Dr. Kass of my plan to paint a red line on my stomach and write, using a magic marker, "No cutting above this line." The hard bargaining came next.

"Don't forget," I reminded him, "that you promised to save my ovaries if possible. I realize that the uterus must go, but not the cervix; that's nonnegotiable."

"What about the appendix?" he asked. "We usually snip it off since we're already in there, and it could flare up in the future."

"I have no problem with that. Since I feel no personal attachment to the appendix," I responded with a straight face, "as far as I'm concerned, you may wear it on your lapel." Satisfied now that the bargaining was over, I patiently awaited his reply.

"No, thanks!" responded Dr. Kass.

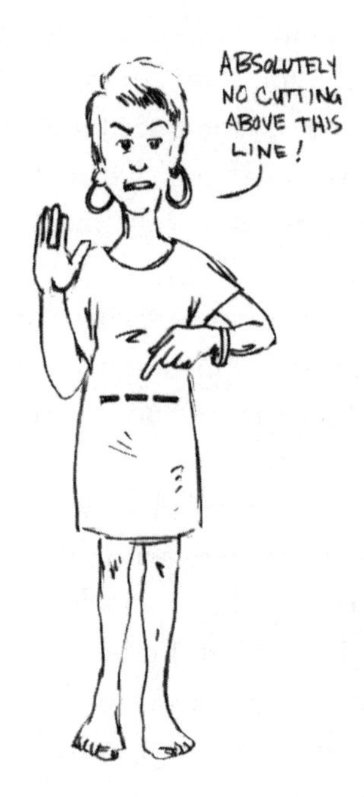

ALSO A FEW days before my surgery, I had routine blood tests and an electrocardiogram (EKG) to evaluate heart function done at the hospital—standard procedure for presurgical patients. A urinalysis may, in some situations, also be required.

A complete blood count (CBC) analyzes the blood not only for the red and white blood cells but also for a platelet count. A sufficient platelet count is necessary to ensure proper clotting.

Some hospitals also require serology testing as part of their preoperative workup. This studies the serum of the blood, analyzing it for antibodies, immune complexes, and antigen-antibody reactions. Focusing on the latter, a rapid plasma reagin (RPR) or venereal disease research laboratory (VDRL) test is included to screen for syphilis.

In addition to these routine tests, my hospital had a pre-admittance check-in policy—a big advantage. I completed all necessary paperwork ahead of time, therefore avoiding additional stress on the day of admittance. Health insurance was verified, a patient information questionnaire was filled out, and consent forms for both surgery and anesthesia were signed. With this taken care of in advance, I would be able to go directly to my room on the morning of surgery as well as leave directly at the time of discharge without needing to first check in at the hospital records office.

Another aspect of my preoperative preparation involved deciding on the type of anesthesia (see the box "Terms to Understand" and the glossary). I had three options to choose from: general anesthesia, spinal block, or an epidural. Of the three Dr. Kass preferred a general anesthesia because he felt it was easier and better for both the doctor and the patient. He explained that when a patient is under a general anesthesia, the body is relaxed and it's easier for the surgeon to cut through relaxed muscle and tissue. The patient experiences nothing, does not awaken before entering the recovery room, and usually remembers nothing before being wheeled back to her room. However, he suggested I consult further with the attending anesthesiologist.

I did phone the anesthesiologist, because like many children who had grown up in the fifties, I had a frightening experience with ether. At the age of twelve I had a minor accident but received a compound fracture of my right wrist. The orthopedic surgeon who was then on call decided to put me to sleep before resetting the fracture. I remember a mask being clamped over my mouth and becoming very frightened and gasping for air. The next day I couldn't figure out why my tongue was so swollen and sore. It was not until many years later that I was told the truth: that I had gone into convulsions and to prevent me from swallowing my tongue, the doctor had grabbed hold of the tongue with a pair of forceps.

Although ether is no longer used, the experience had been so vividly implanted in my mind that the fear of dying in the OR while under anesthesia became painfully real. Not until I began my research did I discover that fear of death is common among presurgical patients, mainly stemming from a sense of loss of total control when under a general anesthesia.

Not until I began my research did I discover that fear of death is common among presurgical patients, mainly stemming from a sense of loss of total control when under a general anesthesia.

Nevertheless, the hospital anesthesiologist agreed with Dr. Kass by encouraging me to go with a general anesthesia for abdominal surgery even though the final decision would be mine. "A sedative beforehand will have a calming effect," he said. "This way, by the time you're wheeled into the operating room, you'll neither feel nor remember a thing. It's very peaceful and there's no trauma." General anesthesia is administered through an IV and is calming because the patient usually remembers nothing before going to sleep. This was my experience.

Both spinal block and epidural create a regional block, and the patient is awake although cannot feel pain. Sometimes it becomes necessary to administer a general anesthetic even after the local was first tried. However, those people who dread the loss of consciousness may prefer this method. This way, it is also possible to keep a watchful eye on the doctor and "assist" the surgeon.

TERMS TO UNDERSTAND

Epidural—An epidural is an injection of an agent into the space surrounding the spinal canal.

General anesthesia—Any anesthesia associated with loss of consciousness is called general anesthesia.

Spinal block—A spinal block is the freezing of the lower part of the body by inserting a needle into the spinal column, which can be painful.

Nevertheless, it did not take me long to decide on general anesthesia because I figured I'd have to deal with enough pain after surgery. Why, then, go through a possible trauma by actually observing it? For me, it made no sense. My greatest fear was that I would fail to wake up after the operation, but then I realized that general anesthesia was, perhaps, the safest way to go. If it would make Dr. Kass's job easier, then why not cooperate? Furthermore, the possibility of first having a local and then a general was somewhat unnerving.

MY MIND and body preparation was coming to a close. The day before surgery I bought a few books that I thought might be enjoyable reading for the hospital and help pass the time. I also purchased a supply of thank-you notes to have on hand to respond to all those individuals who would help me during my recovery.

That evening I packed my overnight case, remembering to take only essential items and *no* valuables. Included were two comfortable nightgowns, a robe, slippers (with traction), toiletries, and a small bag of cosmetics. Besides books, I also took a small address/telephone book plus a little notebook with blank paper for notations, messages—anything I didn't want to forget and would need to jot down.

THERE ARE many ways of coping with presurgical nerves and anxiety. You can meditate, pray, spend time with loved ones, go on a trip, keep really busy, or even start a new hobby. My way was through self-empowerment (studying about hysterectomy, planning for the surgery and its aftermath, taking control where I could) and humor. If you can laugh, or simply experience delight, it not only eases your anxiety but also puts others at ease, too.

Think about those times when you have burst into laughter or had a giggle. Those were the times when you were able to step back from your everyday life concerns and see things from a different perspective. You laugh at a punch line to a joke because of its unexpected perspective on the story line, or you smile with delight when you share a child's wonderment. Every moment provides you with another opportunity to experience life with freshness, delight, and humor. Can you appreciate the moment?

Another source of presurgical nerves or anxiety is feeling intimidated, for a variety of reasons. You may think that you have too many questions, that your questions sound stupid, or that your doctor has better things to do than talk to you. Untrue! You are important, and your questions and concerns are important, too.

If you feel intimidated by all the information you receive in the doctor's office, you can try a couple of tricks. First, ask a relative or a friend to come with you, someone you can trust to explain or review the information you missed. Or, bring an audiotape player to your appointment and record the conversation. You can listen to the tape when you feel calmer, writing down your questions while you are reviewing the tape.

Later in this book you will learn how other women coped with preparing for hysterectomy. What's important to remember is that we all have choices within our respective, unique situations. Do what's best for *you*.

CHAPTER FIVE

THE DAY *of* SURGERY

MY ALARM clock was ringing. It was 5:00 in the morning. Slowly, I got myself up and out of bed as I moved toward the bathroom to shower and get dressed to go to the hospital. This was the morning of surgery. I wasn't nervous. Everything had been done ahead of time so I could afford to feel calm and relaxed.

When I stepped out of the shower, Marty was just getting up, but it was still too early in the morning for us to carry on a conversation. We dressed in silence.

I grabbed my overnight bag, and we went downstairs to feed our two cats and leave for the hospital. It was now 5:45 A.M., and check-in time was in fifteen minutes. The hospital was only a ten-minute drive from our house, so we had allowed plenty of time to get there.

As Marty and I walked into the main entrance of Highland Park Hospital, we were greeted by Mother and Dad, who had already been waiting fifteen minutes. We checked in with the hospital receptionist, who directed us to the second-floor surgical wing where I was assigned a room.

Initially, I had requested a semiprivate room because my insurance would fully cover it, but Marty suggested we go the extra $35 per day for a single room. From personal experience he knew how important it was to have privacy following major surgery, for many reasons: (1) you aren't forced to deal with another person when you want rest; (2) you can focus on your own situation without constant interruptions from a roommate's postsurgical discomforts involving doctors and nurses coming and going; (3) you don't need to share bathroom facilities—a *big* advantage after abdominal surgery since much time is spent in the bathroom; (4) private telephone calls remain private; and, finally, (5) visitors can be many, few, or none—without fear of bothering someone else or of being bothered. For many people, however, a semiprivate room is sufficient.

> *If you feel that someone is behaving in a neglectful, irresponsible, or unprofessional manner, please speak up!*

Some women also stress the desire for private nurses, but this was not an important consideration for me because the nursing staff at Highland Park Hospital was not only outstanding but very attentive—so much so that I found myself wanting to thank each one personally with a note after being discharged.

The point is that you should feel comfortable with the numerous professionals who care for you during your stay in the hospital. If you feel that someone is behaving in a neglectful, irresponsible, or unprofessional manner, please speak up! First, make your concerns known to the head nurse. If the problem persists, contact the hospital's risk management department. If you cannot advocate for yourself, ask a friend or relative to act on your behalf.

WHILE I changed into a hospital gown from my street clothes, Marty and the folks waited outside my room for a few minutes before rejoining me. Then began a whirlwind of activity.

Nurses came and went. Dr. Kass greeted me, followed by the anesthesiologist, whom I later learned was from France. I had already agreed to the general anesthetic and was grateful for his suggestion of a sedative. I saw Ellen, Dr. Kass's nurse, at the door, and she was smiling as she entered the room. She had been granted permission to observe my surgery. Knowing that she would be with me in the operating room, I felt serenely confident. Although this may seem illogical, Ellen and I had been friends for many years, and I felt that if she were with me in the OR, I'd survive! Besides, I had taken the time to do my homework very thoroughly by researching hysterectomies, organizing the house, and getting myself into the best possible shape—physically and mentally. Everything was under control.

As soon as the doctors and Ellen had left to scrub for surgery, a male nurse entered to administer the sedative.

"Which side do you want to face?" he asked. Looking at my parents and Marty, I bashfully turned to face Mom and Dad while exposing my bare bottom to Marty and the nurse. Then I lay back to relax and wait for the drug to take effect.

Soon I began feeling strangely calm. Before long, two orderlies came in to transfer me from my bed to a waiting gurney that would take me into the OR. Marty, Mother, and Dad were permitted to walk alongside the cart as I was wheeled down the hall, and then they kissed me good-bye at the OR entrance.

"If I live through this, I'm going to write a book!" Those were my parting words, and that's all I remember.

I was told later that as soon as I saw Ellen standing in the OR, I thanked her profusely for being there. I also thanked Dr. Kass for arranging to have her present during the surgery. Then, just before the anesthesiologist put me to sleep, he leaned over toward me and softly said, "*Bon nuit,* Nancy." I was asleep in seconds, and the surgery began.

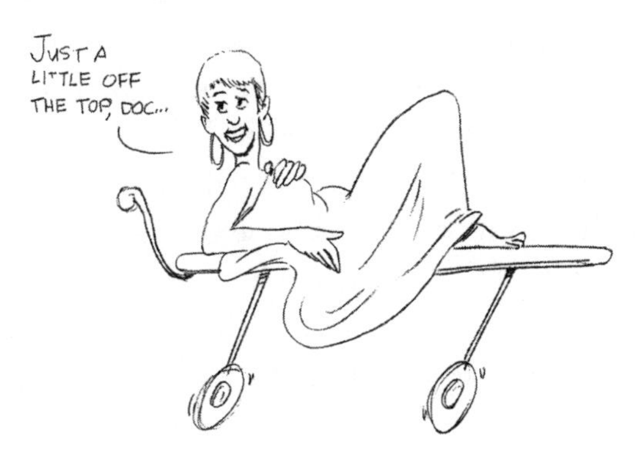

CHAPTER SIX

IN *and* OUT *of the* HOSPITAL

TUESDAY, DAY 1

While being wheeled back to my hospital room from recovery, I babbled incessantly as I was emerging from sedation.

"Do I have cancer? Did they take out my ovaries? Both? Oh, no! Why? What about the cervix? They saved a piece of it? Which piece? How big?" I clung to my husband's hand. "I love you, Marty. Please, don't leave me alone here. I'm so afraid."

I saw Mom and Dad. I was told they had all been waiting several hours to see me while I was in surgery, then recovery. Mother was holding a beautifully decorated mug from her and Dad that was filled with delicate flowers.

Fading in and out of consciousness I lay half awake, barely aware of the telephone ringing. Dad was speaking with my boss when a phone call came from my friend Lois. I am told I carried on a twenty-minute conversation with her but don't remember anything. Nor do I remember the call from my son Rob.

A few minutes later I received a call from Yuri, a dear friend with whom I had formed a strong bond several years prior. He had been a "refusenik" (a Soviet Jew who had been denied his legal right to emigrate from the former USSR), and I had conducted a national rescue effort to free him. We later published two books, each detailing our single experience but written from our own distinct perspective.[1] He had been very worried and wanted to know I was all right. Yuri had just called me at home the day before surgery to wish me good luck and now was one of the very first to call on the day of surgery and the very first with whom I remember speaking. I was groggy, unaware, and disoriented. I spoke with him in a raspy voice that seemed different from my own. Yet, a gradual and wonderful awareness began making its way through the mental fog: my good friend, Yuri, cared about me.

The incision was uncomfortable, but most painful of all was the gas. I had forgotten from my reading that after abdominal surgery the belly is swollen with gas and hurts! Two tubes remained inside me from surgery: a catheter attached to my bladder, and an intravenous tube that pumped nourishment and antibiotics into my body through a needle inserted into a vein on the back of my hand. My mouth was dry; a few blisters existed on my bottom lip, which was also swollen; and I felt a small canker sore on the side of my tongue. These were minor discomforts that stemmed from the breathing tube that had been inserted down my throat during surgery.

I was very thirsty and kept asking for something to drink, but all I received was a piece of crushed ice or a damp washcloth to moisten my parched mouth. No matter how much I complained, the medical staff wouldn't budge on this issue. Not even a sip of water was I permitted on that first day because they feared it could make me nauseous. As I lay there motionless, I enjoyed the comfort of my family.

Very shortly my doctor came to tell me everything had gone very well although there had been a surprise. In addition to the tumor, which had grown somewhat larger since the tests had been taken at the beginning of the summer, I also had endometriosis. I remembered reading about this condition in my medical books but had glossed over those pages because I felt the material was irrelevant to my situation (see Chapter 2). Nevertheless, my body cavity had been filled with dried blood that resembled piles of dark brown mud. This condition had escaped both the ultrasound and the MRI because of the size and density of the fibroid tumor.

I searched for reasons why I had developed endometriosis; perhaps I had it because it often strikes women who lead an active life. Now I could acknowledge that I did indeed fall into that category. Throughout my forties life was unusually exciting, but very stressful. I was working both nationally and internationally in trying desperately to win Yuri's freedom from the former Soviet Union. A long, hard struggle ensued while we fought from both sides of the Iron Curtain for his freedom and right to emigrate. My emotions were up and down—exhilarated by challenge and international intrigue, frightened with worry for Yuri and his family, burdened by the awesome responsibility, and too often depressed. The entire three years that Yuri spent as a political prisoner (a prisoner of conscience) in a Siberian labor camp were a time of deep anguish and round-the-clock monitoring. Rest and relaxation were an unfamiliar experience at that time. Therefore, unbeknownst to me, I had been in a high-risk category for developing endometriosis.

"Nancy," said Dr. Kass, "either you have an unusually high tolerance for pain, or you've been in excruciating discomfort for some time and have not said anything." Naturally I was surprised to learn about this additional problem. Although I had been uncomfortable and had experienced painful cramps, I didn't stop to think it could be anything other than the tumor that was bearing down on my bladder and displacing other organs such as the intestines. Having carried two pregnancies to term, I had reasoned that a tumor the size of a grapefruit was indeed smaller than a full-term fetus and would not push my internal organs out of place any more than a normal pregnancy. Moreover, I had decided, in advance, not to make an issue of any pain or discomfort for fear that someone in my family might become unnecessarily alarmed and march me off to the hospital for immediate surgery.

Much later I recalled the difficulty the technician had during the ultrasound in trying to get a clear picture of both my uterus and ovaries. Instead of the usual sharp image, the pictures appeared gray and fuzzy. In retrospect, this should have been a clue that some type of foreign material might have been present to obstruct the view. Had I known about this additional problem, it probably would have influenced my decision on moving up the date for surgery.

Ellen came in. I was so happy to see her again, especially after surgery! It had been very interesting for her to be present in the OR, especially to observe her two bosses, Dr. Kass and Dr. Harry Burstein, while performing their "best work." Dr. Burstein, an associate of Dr. Kass who was also the chairman of the department of obstetrics and gynecology at Highland Park Hospital, assisted Dr. Kass in surgery. "They were so focused," she later exclaimed. As a nurse working with pregnant moms, Ellen has frequently been present in the delivery room to help coach her patients. She is a compassionate, perceptive medical professional with a fervor for learning. Her first opportunity to observe a hysterectomy in progress was mine. As her close friend, I was delighted to give her this unique gift! Also, I think it was important to me personally that she would be there to witness the procedure when I could not. She had been my "watchful eyes."

Although this first day was long and tiring, I was so groggy that it didn't seem to matter. Speaking was somewhat difficult because the surgical breathing tube had irritated my throat, yet that didn't stop me from talking! Raspy voice and all, I chatted incessantly all day and all night with anyone willing to listen. I did notice, however, that I was forgetting words as well as my place in conversation. Someone had to remind me. If I stopped speaking to answer the telephone or to greet someone who had just entered my room, I did not have a

Although this first day was long and tiring, I was so groggy that it didn't seem to matter. Speaking was somewhat difficult because the surgical breathing tube had irritated my throat, yet that didn't stop me from talking!

clue as to what we had been discussing prior to the interruption. If I did not concentrate on what I was saying, with or without interruptions, I would lose my train of thought. Nevertheless, I wasn't needlessly upset because the doctor had warned me of this possibility beforehand, a result of the anesthesia. He had said the problem could continue for several days until all traces of anesthesia had left my body. I made a joke out of missing words. "It's gone," I'd say. "What was I talking about? OK, I'm waiting for the green light. There it is, I remember!"

I was fortunate to have various visits and phone calls from friends that first day, although I was very groggy. One friend brought me a beautiful azalea plant filled mostly with buds, but one pink flower had symbolically opened. She told me to watch the plant each day as buds bloomed and new ones formed, that it would be a sign of my daily recovery. Soon, she said, the flowers would be in full bloom and I would be as good as new.

Now, as I found myself once again surrounded by immediate family, I felt their warmth and love. That entire first day Marty, Mom, and Dad sat vigil at my bedside. Knowing they were there was greatly comforting to me. When I wanted to say something, they listened. Mostly they let me rest. My spirits soared when my son, Steve, and his wife, Sherri, came to see me. Only Rob was missing since he lived out of town.

Suddenly I realized the lateness of the hour and suggested that the kids go for dinner. I knew they must be hungry after a long work day. Winking at Sherri, I told her about some nice "Chardonnay" under my bed if she were interested in a cocktail before supper. Knowing that I was referring to the clear plastic bag attached to my catheter tube, her appropriate response was, "Yuck!"

Once everyone had left I tried to sleep, but it was difficult. The night nurse rearranged my pillows for my head, back, and stomach to give me added support and comfort, and the foot of the bed was raised to elevate my legs. When I felt pain, I was instructed to push a button to release a small amount of Demerol that entered my body through the intravenous tube. I could not overmedicate myself because if I pushed the button more than once every ten minutes, a safety shut-off valve was activated. I dozed fitfully. In the middle of the night I awakened with my first hot flash. Because I had arrived at the hospital that morning on the last day of my menstrual cycle, it was indeed a shock to experience what I had feared were night sweats that first evening. Depressing? Oh, yes! Later, I realized that flushes are a common side effect of Demerol.

WEDNESDAY, DAY 2

Morning came, along with nurses, doctors, telephone calls, and visitors. Breakfast arrived, my first meal since the night before surgery, but it was unappetizing because I was permitted only a liquid diet. Breakfast consisted of red Jell-O, red fruit-flavored ice, juice, chicken broth, and tea. I picked at it, then sent it back practically untouched.

Mom and Dad returned to keep me company. They sat reading while I tried hard to concentrate on the daily newspaper, but I soon gave up and resorted to working crossword puzzles. The television was on, too, but kept at low volume. Its only purpose: an added distraction.

Lunch was delivered—the same selection of food as breakfast, except a different color. Instead of red, lunch was yellow. I worried that dinner might be pea green.

Yuri phoned again that afternoon. He wanted to know whether I had followed his presurgical instructions by informing the doctor of my "need" for a second catheter. I admitted I had not. He became upset with me. Although I understood his concern regarding abdominal surgery, the inability to pass gas, I had felt it better to leave this issue up to Dr. Kass. Nevertheless, Yuri's thinking differed sharply on this subject. Many years ago he had undergone gall bladder surgery in Moscow and remembered all too well the problems with abdominal surgery. Not being able to void *is* painful, but if another tube was not suggested by my own physician, I wasn't interested.

Just then, a friend appeared from the hall carrying a large box. Inside I discovered a beautiful white gown. What could be more feminine than a luscious new gown for a gal who had just lost all her internal female parts, and was lying there prone in a hospital bed? Immediately I rang for the nurse to help me into it.

First, a sponge bath. How amazingly clean and fresh it can make a woman feel, just one day after surgery. Afterwards, the nurse gently helped me into the new ensemble, carefully avoiding my connecting tubes and *voilà!* I felt almost feminine again.

Later that day another nurse tried to help me stand and take my first steps. Good postoperative care requires patients to get up and move about as soon as possible to prevent blood clots from forming in the legs. Walking also helps the system get moving again for both bladder and bowel control. Nevertheless, I was too dizzy and nauseous to comply. She tried to raise me to a sitting position, but I knew the attempt would be futile and told her so. I was afraid that if I stood, I'd black out and collapse.

"My chest hurts," I complained as she turned to leave. "I don't understand it."

"Of course, Nancy. It's because of the endometriosis. They had to clean you out and then repositioned everything back inside of you."

"What?" I asked, taken aback by the announcement. "You mean, like rearranging furniture in a room?"

"Exactly," she replied, missing the implied humor.

"Remind me to ask Dr. Kass for the new floor plan," I responded, still chuckling.

Early that evening Marty rejoined me. Our friends Herb and Helene also came, followed by my sister Linda and her friend Jerry. Just eight days earlier Jerry himself had been sprung from the hospital following difficult surgery. The topic of conversation: surgery, and its aftermath. "Ohhh," I thought disheartedly, "might this be an indication of the next stage of life—when talk seems focused on illness and decay?"

Soon after Linda and Jerry had left, I suddenly felt the urge to go to the bathroom because the catheter had been removed earlier that day and I was now on my own.

In my soft and raspy voice I whispered, "I've got to go to the bathroom." No one heard. Struggling to sit up a little more, I said, with great urgency, "I have to go pee."

This time, Marty immediately rose to his feet and rushed over to help me up. However, I was practically dead weight inasmuch as I could not move a muscle on my own without pain. Moreover, I was attached to the intravenous equipment.

"What should I do?" he asked, looking helpless.

"Please," I said, "disconnect the equipment from the wall so I can get up. You'll have to push it behind me."

Herb then got up from his chair to assist Marty. With my husband supporting one arm and Herb the other they carefully escorted me into the bathroom while Helene brought up the rear by guiding my "life support" equipment to which I was attached by the intravenous tube. It's not easy to fit four people and one bulky piece of equipment into a tiny hospital bathroom. Once inside, Marty tried to gently lift the back of my gown so I could sit down. I stared at him in horror.

"What are you doing?" I asked.

"I'm trying to help you, honey," he replied looking pained.

"Please," I said, "go out and let me be. Close the door behind you, and I'll tell you when I'm finished."

"But," said Marty, trying so hard to be thoughtful, "I'm afraid you might faint."

"Marty, I'll faint if you stay. Please."

The three of them then quietly exited my small cubicle, leaving me inside with my feeding tubes and some privacy. Then, I was led back to bed by my three bodyguards.

Walking was terribly uncomfortable. I was unable to stand up straight because of the pain from my stitches, and my stomach felt so heavy, almost as if it might drop to the floor.

Dr. Burstein came by to inquire how I was feeling.

"Hungry," I replied. "I don't like the liquid diet and would prefer real food."

"Sorry," said he. "Not until you pass gas."

"But, Doctor, I can't do it if I don't first eat something."

"Oh, yes, you can," he said.

I was encouraged to cough as much as possible not only to dislodge the phlegm but also to help keep the lungs expanded, which would prevent pneumonia and fever.

"But, Doctor, do you think that might be possible by Friday?"

"I can't say for certain, Nancy," he stated matter-of-factly.

Looking him squarely in the eye and with a very straight face I said, "Doctor, you know that Friday is Shabbat and I'm a very religious person. I can't have dinner without a glass of wine."

Shaking his head, Dr. Burstein slowly replied, "Then you need a glass of red wine, right?"

"That's right, Doctor."

"No! Not until you first pass gas and void." Without saying another word he turned and moved toward the door, winked, and quickly departed.

After everyone had left for the night, I tried to sleep but every time I moved a muscle my abdomen hurt. If I coughed to bring up phlegm from surgery, I experienced sharp pains around the incision. Yet, I was encouraged to cough as much as possible not only to dislodge the phlegm but also to help keep the lungs expanded, which would prevent pneumonia and fever. Coughing also helps rid the body of gas. Following any kind of abdominal surgery the belly becomes distended with gas and can be excruciatingly painful, sometimes more so than the incision itself. The afternoon nurse had instructed me on how to firmly hold a pillow over my abdomen when I coughed, which would help reduce the pain.

Sometime in the middle of the night I rang for the nurse to help me again into the bathroom. As I sat there trying to void, I suddenly burst into tears. I was crying with my entire being. Not only was I emotionally distraught, but physically it seemed that my body was urgently expressing some primal response to the trauma of having been injured. I mourned for my precious female parts, sitting in a bottle of formaldehyde, downstairs in the hospital laboratory, waiting to be dissected. Although I knew it was ridiculous, I suddenly wanted them back. Reattached!

It is common to feel depressed after surgery, especially following a hysterectomy. Loss of parts of the body can be very distressing for most people, and even more difficult for some when those lost parts are internal. It's easier to accept what is gone when you can see it. Many therapists equate a posthysterectomy depression to a postpartum depression. Although it's usually a temporary condition, the manifesting repercussions from this surgery can be upsetting because a hysterectomy plays havoc on a woman's system. The ability to cry acts as an important part of the healing process as it releases tension and expresses deep resultant emotion. Women, therefore, should not try to hold back and suppress their sadness. It is natural to feel sad.

Finally, I dried my eyes and said sternly to myself, "Come on, Nancy, get on with it. You don't need those parts anymore. You'll be OK. You've survived other traumas. You'll survive this, too." With that, I dried my eyes and was all right, at least for the time being.

THURSDAY, DAY 3

"Good morning," said the nurse as she came in to check my vital signs. "Did you get any sleep?"

"No. It was impossible. My incision hurts, the gas pains are uncomfortable, and I tried to go to the bathroom but was unsuccessful."

"Don't worry," said she. "You're doing miraculously well. Why, you were just operated on two days ago, and already you're walking around. Why don't you push the Demerol button and get some pain relief?"

"I'm trying to do without pain killers, if possible, because it makes me dizzy and nauseous."

"Don't be so valiant, Nancy. You've hardly used any at all, and it's here to make you feel better."

With that, she gave me a dose of Demerol. When you first push the button, nothing happens immediately, but then you feel a sharp burning sensation in the back of your hand a few seconds later when the Demerol begins to course through your vein at the point where the intravenous needle has been inserted. Then, the pain begins to subside.

"Your breakfast tray will be here shortly," she reminded me.

"Breakfast? Will I have real food today?" I asked hopefully.

"No, I'm afraid not. Not until you void."

"OK," I said, "then as of 7:00 this morning I'm declaring a hunger strike. You know the story: the operation was a success but the patient died. Well, let it be on your conscience that this was a postsurgical death by starvation," I said.

One hour later the breakfast tray arrived. Red liquids!

"No!" I shouted, although my voice could still barely be heard above a faint whisper.

I had been reading Cornelia Otis Skinner's book *Sarah Bernhardt* and had just finished the part where Sarah first lands in America with her entourage from Paris. No sooner did she disembark ship than she was met by an "obnoxious" American man who publicly insulted her, then further delighted in her misery. After the insult this same man sent two dozen long-stemmed red roses to her hotel on a weekly basis, which she perceived as a gesture of mockery and threw them out the window.

Remembering Sarah Bernhardt, I told the woman who had delivered the tray, "If you insist upon leaving that tray of liquid substance, I'll just throw it out the window."

The poor woman looked quite forlorn until Dr. Kass, at that precise moment, stepped into my room.

"You're looking much better this morning, Nancy," said he. "I think we'll start you on soft foods today."

I shot him a quick sigh of relief, as the woman with the tray made a quiet exit.

Next came the best news of all. Dr. Kass informed me that the pathology report had just come back from the lab—negative. No cancer!

I had some nice visits with friends during the day, although at times I felt giddy. At the time, however, I didn't realize that my giddiness was the result of a sudden hormonal imbalance caused by the surgery. Later in the afternoon I received a call from Yuri.

"Hi, Nancy, how are you feeling?" he asked with genuine concern.

"I'm OK, thank you, Yuri. I'm a little stronger than yesterday, but my belly is still very sore. Yet, there's less pain than yesterday. How are you?"

"Fine, Nancy. I want to ask you something."

"Yuri," I said in a very controlled voice (and a playful gleam of which he was unaware). "I know you have a question for me, but first I want to ask you something." My voice was sounding stronger as I readied myself for the sting. "Did you move your bowels today?" Without pausing for a second to permit him a chance to react, I quickly continued, "and if you did, did everything come out all right? If you'd like to share your experience with me, I'll be happy to share mine with you and we can have a real dialogue." Grinning while enjoying every moment, I awaited his response.

Dead silence. My friend, the distinguished Russian scientist, was indeed a very private person. Suddenly, Yuri exploded into peals of laughter until he finally was able to catch his breath and reply.

"That's OK, Nancy. Now I know you're back to normal."

From that moment on, I knew we'd have no further discussion regarding my bowel and bladder functions. These would remain a private matter.

EARLY THAT evening Marty returned. He was dressed in shorts and a T-shirt, all set for his tennis match later that night. After a busy day he looked tired and drawn. Poor guy. He was assuming all my responsibilities on top of running to the hospital to see me. Already after three days this new routine appeared to be taking its toll.

Later that evening I tried to rest. I snapped on the TV and opened my book, but couldn't concentrate. I reflected on some of the visits I had had that day. Earlier in the day the hospital dietician had come in to see me. She was very lovely and even told me about her own experience with surgery some twenty-five years earlier. "It was interesting," said she, "because you really find out who your friends are. Most of them called and were supportive, but a few never even bothered picking up the telephone to see how I was doing." I thought about her words, and I was filled with sadness.

Suddenly a rather young and odd-looking man, short and small in stature, appeared in the doorway. He was dressed in an ill-fitting black suit with curly black hair, black beard and mustache, and small wire-framed spectacles perched awkwardly on the bridge of his nose. I noticed the yarmulke pinned to the back of his head and realized he must be an Orthodox rabbi.

"Mrs. Rosenfeld?" he inquired, not venturing any further into the room than the outer doorway, but just poking his head inside.

"Yes," I responded, curiously.

With that he quickly fumbled inside his pocket and pulled out a small, crumbled-up piece of paper that he held unsteadily beneath the bridge of his nose. Reading from his notes, he said rapidly in a well-rehearsed, high-pitched voice,

"I'm here to see all the Jews and wish you a speedy recovery. Nice to meet you. Bye!"

Those eighteen words recited, and he was out the door in a flash! For a moment I lay there immobilized. Speechless. Then, my eyes welled up with tears as shrieks of laughter poured freely out. I clutched my sore abdomen because every time I laughed the pain became excruciating. Yet, I was convulsed and unable to stop no matter how painful it was. Immediately, I grabbed for the telephone receiver. I needed to reach someone quickly. My emotions were raw and overwhelming me. The only one I knew for sure would be home at that very moment was Mother. Fumbling with the phone, I dialed.

"Mother! Hear this!"

Somehow, laughing and crying simultaneously, I managed to relate what had just occurred. I spoke breathlessly, too rapidly, yet she managed to hear. Mother listened patiently.

"Yes," she admitted with reserve, that it was indeed one of the most bizarre episodes she could recall hearing. Then, "Nancy, are you OK?" she asked woefully.

LATER THAT night when Dr. Kass stopped by while making his rounds, I told him about the incident. He, too, chuckled. But neither he nor mother seemed to think the event as funny as I. Then I informed him about Dr. Burstein not permitting me any wine because I had not successfully "passed gas." Right then and there he decided that a small glass of white wine would do me no damage, so he personally went to take care of it. He expressed concern about my being so emotionally volatile and felt the glass of wine might even help. What's more, he promised to put me on a regular hospital diet beginning in the morning. For that I thanked him profusely.

Once he had left and my wine had been delivered, I again tried to rest. Before retiring for the night, I went into the bathroom to brush my teeth and wash up. Then I snapped off the light, closed my eyes, and waited for slumber. Nothing happened. My mind was busy, very busy; my body, restless.

I soon gave up and went for a walk. With effort, I paced back and forth along the hospital corridor as the nurses had been encouraging me to do. I was reminded to stand up straight.

"No slouching, Nancy," I'd hear a nurse say as we passed each other in the hall.

"Don't be afraid. You won't burst your stitches." Nodding in response, I attempted to straighten my back while grasping my stomach for support. It hurt, but I was told that standing would not get easier if I didn't straighten up. All at once, I had a flashback of balancing books on top of my head as a teenager—a lesson in good posture. Enough of this. Two or three laps up and down the hall seemed more than sufficient. I was becoming impatient, edgy. Tired and bored, I started for my room.

I heard the elderly woman on the other side of the wall who was obviously in the bathroom. The poor dear was groaning and moaning and throwing up, just as I had been doing only two days earlier. Then I returned to my bedroom, where I hoped to find some peace and quiet. No sooner did I rearrange my pillows and gently ease myself back into bed when I heard the elderly man on the other side of my bedroom wall begin to shout.

"Help! Nurse! My tubes just fell out and I'm hemorrhaging. I think I'm bleeding to death!"

That call was followed by instant commotion in the hallway just outside his door. Yet, I thought, "My God, that poor dear man if that is really true. . . .

"But, what on earth am *I* doing on a floor like this with all these sick people who are moaning and groaning and screaming and throwing up while I, too, have just undergone major surgery?" Yet I was able to maintain my sense of humor. What's wrong with these people? I had to escape, quickly! I was afraid my life had shrunk to the size of this hospital room. Both my mind and my emotions were getting out of control. "Focus, Nancy, focus," I heard my alter ego saying. "What's your goal? What do you need?"

I attempted to straighten my back while grasping my stomach for support. It hurt, but I was told that standing would not get easier if I didn't straighten up.

It was then that I made up my mind to speak with the doctor during his morning rounds about being discharged. I rang for the nurse to request a sedative so I might sleep. Before handing me the requested drug, she first took my temperature and discovered I had a low fever. I knew that meant trouble for a morning release but yet was determined not to worry about it. I had to get out. I was dying to get out—no, I would die if I did not get out. Of this I was convinced! Yet postoperative fevers can be a sign of infection, and, in rare cases, an abscess, which means trouble. Whatever the problem, for my own sanity and peace of mind, I needed to get home to rest and recuperate in familiar surroundings. Gradually, my eyelids became heavy and I was overcome with sleep.

FRIDAY, DAY 4

I slept poorly because of the fever and also because of being painfully bloated and sore from surgery. As I lay waiting for the doctor to enter, I felt anxious about going home and mentally rehearsed what I wanted to say. I expected him early.

Dr. Kass appeared even before my breakfast tray was delivered.

"Good morning, Doctor," I said, feigning a stoic expression. "I know what you're going to say. Either you'll evict me for disturbing the peace because I've been laughing uproariously, or you'll hold me hostage for another twenty-four hours because I've got a fever and haven't been able to pass gas. But," I paused, readying for the punch, "if you don't release me, I'll flee—right down the fire escape."

Shaking his head with wonder while maintaining a quizzical grin, he replied earnestly,

"I don't want to hold you hostage, but I can't set you free with a temperature, either. Let's see how you're doing this afternoon. If the fever goes down, I'll release you tonight," he promised. After checking the incision to make sure it was properly healing, he removed all the staples while distracting me in conversation. I didn't even realize he was removing them until after he'd finished. When he showed me the staple remover, I counted sixteen used staples.

Then he pulled up a chair next to my bed.

"Let's discuss hormone therapy. We're going to start you on estrogen today, and you'll be taking a drug called Premarin. Premarin is the only natural form of estrogen, which is actually made from the urine of pregnant horses. All other brands are synthetic."

"What about the estrogen patch?" I asked, turning up my nose at his reference to pregnant horse's urine. The patch, an estrogen-filled bandage usually applied to the buttocks, is replaced every one to three days with a new one. The dosage of estrogen can be regulated by adding more bandages. With this method of ERT the secreted hormone passes through the bandage, entering the skin, and is absorbed into the bloodstream.[2]

"I would rather have you on pills because we have greater flexibility in regulating the dosage. You can't adjust it with the patch. I'm not putting you on progesterone, either, the hormone secreted by the ovaries that helps to stimulate menstrual bleeding, because your uterus has been removed and you don't need it. But, you do have the option of taking testosterone along with estrogen."

Although Dr. Kass commented on the widely publicized debate over the possible linkage between estrogen use and breast cancer, he went on to say that studies so far have found no increase in breast cancer among women taking the hormone.

"Earlier data," continued Dr. Kass, "supported the theory that women were at high risk and could not take HRT because of such reputed factors as: family history of cancer (breast, ovarian, or uterine), strong family history of heart disease, diabetes, high cholesterol or high triglyceride levels of blood fat, and smoking cigarettes.

"Nevertheless, the indications and contraindications for women who cannot take estrogen have been changing over the past five years. At this time the only two *absolute* contraindications are (1) active thrombophlebitis (blood clots) and (2) the recent incidence of breast or uterine cancer. All other contraindications are relative."

For women on estrogen who have retained their uterus, most doctors also advise them on taking progesterone in conjunction with estrogen because it seems to have a counterbalancing effect in preventing endometrial cancer. Women who no longer have a uterus do not need progesterone because endometriosis originates in the uterine lining.

Testosterone, the male sex hormone, is offered to ovariectomized patients who are concerned about a lessened libido as a direct result of their lost ovaries. However, within a few weeks of taking this hormone some women have reported male traits such as hairiness and deepening of the voice. The risk of male characteristics developing is even greater with the use of androgen, the male sex hormone responsible for masculine traits.[3]

"Studies of HRT are still inconclusive," continued Dr. Kass, "but there appear to be more positives than negatives for those women who are eligible. Nonusers of HRT are at greater risk of developing: cardiovascular disease; blood clots; osteoporosis; and overall acceleration of the aging process, particularly relating to skin and muscle tone.

"In fact, Nancy," he said, "there's a study that began in 1982 that is tracking fifty thousand female nurses for the effects of estrogen replacement therapy on their systems. The study will continue forever, and it's possible that these nurses may be able to remain on estrogen throughout their lives. However, current statistics seem to indicate that after the age of sixty there is a 10 to 15 percent increase in the risk factor for developing breast cancer after taking hormones for over ten years. Nevertheless, far more women die annually from heart disease than cancer of the breast or reproductive system."

For women on estrogen who have retained their uterus, most doctors also advise them on taking progesterone in conjunction with estrogen because it seems to have a counterbalancing effect in preventing endometrial cancer. Women who no longer have a uterus do not need progesterone because endometriosis originates in the uterine lining.

Cardiovascular disease is caused by excess amounts of cholesterol, carried through the cardiovascular system in the form of lipoproteins (lipids covered by a protein coat). A *lipid* is a fat or fatlike substance that is normally present in the body. Triglycerides, fatty acid compounds, represent approximately 95 percent of the fat we consume and can be both satrated (from animal sources) and unsaturated (from plant sources). Therefore, a high-saturated-fat diet of meat and dairy is generally also high in cholesterol. Those people with high levels of cholesterol are warned to reduce their saturated fat levels and increase their polyunsaturated fats (any plant and animal fat and oils with a low cholesterol content).

Lipoproteins can be either high density (HDL) or low density (LDL). HDL, considered "good" cholesterol, has a higher concentration of lipoproteins that actually remove cholesterol from the blood vessels and, thereby, decrease the risk of coronary heart disease. LDL, the "bad" cholesterol, is known to deposit excess amounts of cholesterol on the artery walls. I'm able to remember the difference between HDL and LDL by associating "H" with high (the higher the density of lipoproteins, the greater your protection from clogged arteries), and "L" with low (low density is "bad"). Even if your total cholesterol level (HDL plus LDL) is high, the high HDL count, within certain limits, is considered good. HRT helps lower the cholesterol level, thus decreasing a person's risk of cardiovascular disease. Because estrogen-deficient women are at a much higher risk of developing cardiovascular-related problems, many doctors recommend that hysterectomized women follow a regimen of HRT.[4]

After discussing my options and weighing the pros and cons, I asked for Dr. Kass's professional opinion.

"It's entirely your decision," he said, whereupon I decided upon estrogen replacement without testosterone.

I WAS euphoric. I was going home! I couldn't wait to tell Marty, and I longed to be able to lounge at home and sleep in my own bed. I looked forward to working with the computer and its newly installed e-mail.

The telephone rang. It was Marty's brother Neal.

"How are you doing, Nancy?"

"Much better! In fact, you'll be happy to know I'm now potty trained and will no longer need any assistance to go to the bathroom."

He laughed good-naturedly.

"Nancy, where is your husband? I called his office, but no one's seen him today."

Glancing at the clock, I saw it was five minutes to eleven.

"He could be at the health club, or perhaps he's had an accident," I joked. "Last night I threatened to file for divorce, so maybe I scared him to death."

"OK," Neal replied, failing to get a serious response. "But if you hear anything, let him know I'm looking for him."

"Will do."

By the time Marty finally did call, I had just begun to excitedly tell him of my plans to go home before being stopped dead in my tracks.

"Nancy, I had an accident last night and injured my hip."

"What?" I gasped, suddenly frightened and horrified. Five minutes earlier I had been joking about an accident. Now I felt profoundly guilty and was worried sick.

"What happened?" I whispered.

"I tripped and fell, then got up right away because I didn't realize how bad it was until later. I wanted to tell you last night when I called, but you were too wound up."

"Ohhh," said I, feeling very ashamed.

Dr. Kass walked back in a few minutes later to inform me of his decision to spring me that evening. He'd stop by after office hours for a final check and then I'd be free to go.

After phoning Marty back at the office to ask him to fetch me at five o'clock, I began preparing. A real shower felt delicious, and I luxuriated under the delicate spray for several wonderful minutes. Afterwards I put on makeup, for the first time since entering the hospital, and then got dressed in my tennis warm-up suit. These simple activities were the first steps toward feeling human again.

Next, I began packing, taking my empty bag from the armoire, placing it on a chair, and tossing my meager belongings inside—books, dirty clothes, get-well cards, and gifts. When the bag was packed full, I mustered up all my strength and, with the help of momentum, arched my back and swung the bag from the chair to the bed. Flushed from exertion and more than a little shaky, I suddenly realized what I had done.

Oh, my God. The incision! Grabbing my bruised and swollen stomach, I shuffled back to the nurse's station, but this time with no smugness. With pleading eyes and a pained expression, I motioned for one of them to lend me her chair. Startled, she quickly obliged while the others looked on with great concern.

"For goodness sakes, what on earth have you done?" asked the nurse whose chair I had been offered.

"I just picked up my fifty-pound bag (laden with books from family and friends), then realized I'd been instructed not to lift anything greater than ten pounds, maximum!"

I was terrified of internal hemorrhage. I thought they all looked pale as nobody dared to utter a sound for several seconds. My worst fear was that now I couldn't be discharged. I waited to hear the pronouncement of my "sentence."

"Nancy," she said, "everyone is entitled to one demerit. Don't worry. You won't die. Just don't let it happen again because next time you may not be so lucky." When she said this, she looked at me directly in the eyes, sternly, and then her face widened into a warm smile.

With a sigh of relief I returned to my room and reclined on my bed, grateful for my reprieve, content to wait until help arrived.

Marty walked in an hour early, appearing tired and limping. He sat down beside me to wait for the doctor. I told him about my mistake, and he listened silently, shaking his head with obvious disapproval. I also repeated the story to Dr. Kass when he came in to discharge me.

"Nancy," said he at last, looking more amused than upset. "I must remember to check with the anesthesiologist to see what he spiked your anesthesia with to give you such a high. Go home and relax. No more stunts!"

REENTERING THE house was simply ecstasy. Marty took charge by bringing my things inside, making several trips because of my book bag and flowers, while I sat and watched and enjoyed the attention of our two adoring felines who smothered me with wet, sloppy kisses.

Preparation for bed was slow and arduous. As I gingerly removed my clothes, I stared at my reflection in the full-length bathroom mirror for the first time since before surgery. Ugh! My abdomen was extended with gas, and I still looked very pregnant. At least I could see my toes, an improvement from the day before. It now looked more like a three-month pregnancy rather than six months, but my skin was lumpy from the gas. The incision itself looked raw and fiery red, but it was straight, not jagged or puckered. Fortunately there was no evidence of keloids, an overgrowth of scar tissue that appears thick, raised, and red.

As I gingerly removed my clothes, I stared at my reflection in the full-length bathroom mirror for the first time since before surgery. Ugh! My abdomen was extended with gas, and I still looked very pregnant.

Keloids are at least fifteen times more prevalent in dark-skinned people than in those with lighter skin. Although several reasons are cited, the most consistent explanation is that these scars might reflect an abnormality in the way the body metabolizes a hormone vital to skin coloration.

Carefully, I applied vitamin E directly on the incision to help hasten the healing and minimize scarring. This procedure would be followed for months until the wound healed completely. Dr. Kass had promised that the swelling would continue to go down and would leave no stretch marks. Within several weeks the abdomen should return to normal shape, and with exercise later should be firm as ever.

What I had not realized, however, was the advantage of a hospital bed. In those few short days spent at the hospital I had become dependent on the controls that lowered and raised my bed. Now with Marty's help, I slowly eased myself into our bed as he propped me up with pillows for my head and stomach, along with extra pillows to support my back. I found using a study pillow also helpful because it approximated the angle of the hospital bed. Yet, I even missed the side bars that I had used to support my weight while getting up and down. To compensate for the bars, I would need to roll to one side and lift myself up using arm muscles. For added help in sleeping I took a light sedative shortly before "lights out."

Despite these minor troubles in readjusting to the start of my recovery period, nothing beat the simple joy of being in my own house amid familiar surroundings and loved ones. There really *is* no place like home!

CHAPTER SEVEN

RECUPERATION

SATURDAY, my first day home. It was quiet in the house—no nurses buzzing in and out of the room, no patients calling for help; even the telephone was silent. Curled up at my feet were the two sleeping cats, freshly fed. Marty had been awakened earlier to feed them by their gentle but persistent nudging; then he returned to bed. Carefully and very slowly I began to ease myself out of bed, using my arms while supporting my stomach in an effort to soften the pain.

By that time Marty was in the kitchen preparing breakfast. Shortly afterwards he proudly appeared in the doorway with a tray in hand. Breakfast consisted of a vegetable and sausage omelet for two, toasted bagels with jam and margarine, banana cocoa chip cake, orange juice, and coffee. Under his arm, the morning newspaper. I was speechless. We sat together while enjoying the fruits of his labor. The eggs were cooked to perfection, but the irony was that just one week earlier and after thirty years of marriage he still didn't know where to find anything in the house, let alone how to cook.

So began my first week of recovery. Dr. Kass permitted me to walk the stairs once a day, which suited me fine because the computer was upstairs. To ensure proper rest, an impossibility at the hospital, I restricted phone calls and visitors to after 6 P.M. except for my "short list": immediate family and a few close friends. Monitoring calls was easy thanks to the phone answering machine.

Proper rest is mandatory for a speedy, and complete, physical recovery, which is why it is necessary to limit telephone calls and visitors during this initial recovery period. Surgery puts the body through considerable trauma; healing takes time. Not only is it unwise to overdo too soon following major surgery, but it's nearly impossible. The body's normal level of energy has been sapped of strength because it is working very hard to heal from the trauma of the operation. By giving in to signs of fatigue, you can help your body mend instead of fighting the healing process. Be a friend to your body, not an enemy, and listen to your doctor. Take naps!

Because I had finished preparation for recovery before surgery, I now was able to relax while my "team" went to work. Breakfast was stored the night before in a small upstairs refrigerator so I'd be self-sufficient all morning. Juice, milk, cereal, fresh fruit, and coffee became standard breakfast fare. A heating coil for the coffee easily solved reheating problems.

At noon Lois and Helene became my visiting nurses, supplying me with their "meals on wheels" program. They took turns coming over that first week to prepare lunch and bring in the mail while keeping me company. In case I needed anything, someone was on hand for assistance. I looked forward to these visits. Each had been given a set of house keys to let themselves in without my needing to venture downstairs or risk security by leaving the front door unlocked. The keys were theirs to keep in case of accidents, illness, or—sudden death. Although unlikely, major surgery makes you more aware of the possibility. Their lunch trays were always colorfully designed and beautifully garnished. They also checked up on me often by telephone to make sure I was behaving myself. Helene was concerned about my taking naps, reminding me daily that rest is critical for proper healing. If you follow the rules you'll enjoy a complete recovery. If not, your health could be permanently impaired.

Each night when Marty returned home from work, he'd find me ready to join him for the evening. Comfortably but neatly dressed in lounging pajamas, I tried to look perky, not dowdy. Without hesitation, and as if he had been managing the household all his life, he began preparing dinner. I was not permitted to lift a finger. A far cry from our usual lifestyle! More typically he comes home from the office exhausted, changes into a comfortable sweat suit, and collapses into his favorite chair until dinner is ready. But now he assumed a different role. As he set the table, he did it his way—no napkins, and bottles and plastic containers were the norm rather than our more conventionally used serving pieces.

Dinner preparation was made simple by meals needing only to be popped out of the freezer, into the microwave oven, and onto the kitchen table. Within minutes, *voilà!* A complete meal. The summer's project had paid off. Nothing but a salad needed to be made from scratch. Following supper, Marty permitted me to retire to the den while he did dishes.

Occasionally when it became necessary to buy fresh produce or something in the dairy department, Marty took a short list to the grocery store and did the marketing. Amazing what men can learn when left with few options. I'm not sure he had ever even seen the inside of the grocery store before. He also took charge of the laundry and found his way to the cleaners.

Such practical things are an important consideration. Depending on your resources, you might consider hiring household help for the weeks immediately following surgery. However, if your resources are limited, it is still possible

Depending on your resources, you might consider hiring household help for the weeks immediately following surgery. However, if your resources are limited, it is still possible to obtain assistance. Visiting nurses and Meals on Wheels programs are provided by some agencies based on your income.

to obtain assistance. Visiting nurses and Meals on Wheels programs are provided by some agencies based on your income. Your hospital social worker can help you make these arrangements. You might ask a neighbor to pick up a few important items at the grocery store. Your church or synagogue can also supply you with that extra bit of help and support.

A great majority of my recuperation time was devoted to writing. Yet, only in the hospital had I first discovered how well those months of planning and preparation had really paid off. That I could have felt relaxed and happy in a hospital setting was due largely to the emotional strength and peace of mind that I had derived from being mentally well prepared.

If, on the other hand, it is not your nature to plan and prepare, you can still find peace and relaxation while doing those things that bring you pleasure. For example, you may find that reading a good book while listening to music might be just the right diversion. Perhaps you would enjoy a book of crossword puzzles or a large jigsaw puzzle to occupy your time. You may choose an art project, or try caring for new house plants. For those of you who are computer literate or are connected to the Internet, an inexhaustible amount of time can be productively spent while exploring new concepts and ideas, not to mention being connected to the wondrous world of cyberspace. The key is to engage yourself in activities that can provide enjoyment as well as occupy your mind. This, the recovery period, can be a special time—a time to enjoy feeling pampered while indulging in all those pleasures for which there was never enough time.

SOMETIMES, HYSTERECTOMY with bilateral ovariectomy causes a temporary hormonal deficit, which can also upset a woman's body chemistry until she is placed on daily doses of HRT. Surgery is a massive trauma to the system, and the sudden change affects the whole person. Hot flashes and mood changes become instantly apparent.

Women, like myself, who are prone to depression are usually more likely to have hormonal and chemical disturbances following a hysterectomy. For me, bouts of mania can follow depressive episodes, more commonly known as a bipolar disorder (manic depression).

On the other hand, recent evidence supports the theory that laughing can actually boost the immune system by triggering a flood of pleasure-inducing neurochemicals into the brain. Not only does it lower blood pressure, but researchers also say that laughter produces disease-destroying antibodies and T-cells (white blood cells). Because these "killer cells" have been reported to destroy viruses and even tumors, a hearty laugh is good medicine.[1]

Being confronted with major surgery caused me to reflect upon my life on a deeper level, too, becoming even more introspective than my presurgical self. This unleashed an internal struggle, which is something that had been silently plaguing me for many years. When faced with surgery that is threatening to your very self-image, it can have a gut-wrenching effect upon your life. This is what happened to me. It was at this time that I began, very slowly, to reassess my own values and priorities.

Who and what were most important in my life? How did I now see myself, and where did I feel that I belonged? Was I still on track? Or had I somehow deviated from the original path of my journey? I needed to search, to probe deeply, to seek answers.

Had I not become involved in a writing task, it would have been necessary to focus my attention on something else since finding an interesting project after surgery helps ward off moments of the blues.

Nevertheless, I still anguished over the long-term consequences of surgery. Would my skin lose its elasticity? Would I begin to age at a rapid rate? Would my energy level plummet? And, what about my sexual being—was I destined for a life devoid of sexual joy? It was too soon to know the answers to these questions. Although part of me knew this to be true, my other self wanted immediate answers—that everything be clear and certain. My mental anguish remained in the foreground of my experience during those first days into recovery. In the background was the physical discomfort, painful at times, and a body not like the one I had known before surgery. Would this all pass? Would I regain my strength and be able to move around easily again?

Intellectually, I understood that I would recover and that I'd be fine again, but the gnawing, nagging low-grade worry about my womanhood would not let up. Activity was what permitted me to make it through these times of self-doubt. I was also extremely fortunate to have a caring husband, someone with whom I could confide my innermost fears and anxieties. Social supports are essential throughout the hysterectomy process. It is important to develop or have in place a personal support system to help you through this time. If you are unmarried or a person with few friends or family, seek out a support group and attend it regularly. You might also go into therapy, specifically requesting support and guidance with respect to pelvic surgery and related issues. Make sure the therapist is knowledgeable and skilled in dealing with these issues.

BARELY TWO weeks after surgery I stepped on the scale to discover a loss of ten pounds from my presurgical weight—and without daily exercise! I figured it was partly the tumor and whatever else had been removed, but mostly loss of appetite. Whatever the reason, it felt great and I was determined to keep those extra pounds off. I had heard that women often gain weight following a hysterectomy. Because life becomes temporarily sedentary after surgery, it follows that weight can be gained if one's calorie intake remains the same. Usually there's no appetite the first few days, but as you begin feeling better you may start craving food.

Eventually weight did become an issue. A few months after surgery, I began to notice my weight creeping up. Then I became upset. My former dieting habits were no longer working. I regained not only those lost ten pounds but then some. At that point I reevaluated what I had been eating, how much and how often.

The key to reducing weight and/or keeping it off is moderation—moderate activity and moderate food consumption. These concepts are relative and individually determined. They are based on the amounts of activity and food intake to which you have been accustomed as well as the amounts that your body now requires to maintain your present weight.

It was obvious that at my present level of activity (or inactivity!), I had been overindulgent in the food department. In addition, I had been unaware of the big change in metabolism that normally occurs following a hysterectomy. This change affects the whole person, mentally as well as physiologically.

Menopause is a natural aging process that affects all women, usually by the time a woman reaches her midfifties. When a woman goes through normal menopause, she experiences a gradual decrease in levels of estrogen and progesterone. However, hysterectomized women go through this change abruptly, experiencing "instant menopause." This sudden alteration can have a profound impact on a woman's body chemistry.

When a woman goes through normal menopause, she experiences a gradual decrease in levels of estrogen and progesterone. However, hysterectomized women go through this change abruptly, experiencing "instant menopause." This sudden alteration can have a profound impact on a woman's body chemistry.

Because I had always been slender, I was not mindful of my (postsurgical) eating habits even though I should have been. I frequently pigged out on junk food. The postsurgical me, however, discovered that those extra chocolate chip cookies stuck to my ribs, hips, thighs, and belly and were not easily shed by merely skipping a meal here and there. Even cutting back slightly on my normal food regimen was not enough to stop my gradually increasing weight and rid myself of that excess poundage. Part of the problem was due to the decreased amount of activity, which was not directly related to the surgery. When you're off your feet for extended periods of time, swelling can occur. I had become obsessively involved in writing, failing to adhere to a regular exercise routine and thereby finding every excuse in the world not to exercise.

Besides the change of metabolism following surgery, some women also find that ERT adds up to four or five pounds because of fluid retention (although it may self-correct within three months).[2] If fluid retention is a problem, your doctor can easily regulate your dosage of hormones. Taking a mild diuretic and cutting down on salt can also alleviate bloating.

MY ONLY immediate complaint, other than the expected soreness of the abdomen, was some minor pain and swelling in my left hand where the intravenous needle had been inserted. At first I didn't think much about this because it seemed unrelated to surgery. However, after a couple weeks had passed and the hand had not improved, I began taking note. At my two-week postsurgical checkup I questioned my doctor and was informed of a thrombophlebitis, or blood clot—the aftermath of intravenous needle insertion and common for surgical patients. Gradually within a few weeks it would disappear and was nothing dangerous. I was advised to use hot compresses and gently massage the hand to help dissolve the clot more quickly.

At week 3 I was allowed typical extended privileges: walking stairs more than once a day, increasing gradually, and dining out as long as I didn't drive. I also began taking short walks outdoors as well as enjoying the garden I had worked so hard to create before being hospitalized. Heavy housework was still out of the question, but easy tasks were permitted such as light dusting, table setting, helping with dinner dishes, and caring for my animals and plants.

During the fourth week driving was permitted. This activity had been restricted because it poses a great strain on the pelvic muscles besides requiring very alert responses. Swimming, a healing activity, was also added to the acceptable list as long as I did not overdo. If you're not a swimmer, you may enjoy other healing activities such as brisk walking, biking, or even dancing. The main thing to keep in mind is moderation.

"Let your body decide how far you can swim, but no marathons," warned Dr. Kass.

His suggestion: I "play" in the water and use the Jacuzzi, but only a minute or two in the Jacuzzi so I wouldn't become faint from the heat.

That first dip felt splendid. I listened to my body, cautiously swimming one lap and realizing I felt fine. Gradually I increased the number of laps that week, so by the weekend I was up to my normal one-half mile. I now felt as if I was really on that road to recovery.

I believe it's important to exercise self-discipline and not extend the convalescence period too long. If you psych yourself up to feeling normal, you will heal faster. Nevertheless, do not push too far—there remains a fine line between "normal activity" and overdoing. (Some appropriate recovery exercises are described in Chapter 13.)

Dianna, a former fitness instructor, adds that regularity is the key component to a successful fitness program.

"Make a schedule for yourself and keep that commitment," she advises. "Some people mark down their exercise workouts on their appointment calendars so that exercise time is less likely to be preempted by something else.

"Additionally," Dianna says, "people who are just establishing a regular exercise routine should learn to stop exercising before fatigue sets in. If you stop when you feel good, then your body will learn to associate this good feeling with exercise and you'll be more apt to return to it."

Dianna also recommends *not* comparing yourself and your capabilities (or appearance) with anyone else.

"Focus on small steps and slow improvement over weeks, not days," she suggests. "You should be able to see a difference in your physical capacity over a period of weeks; your aim, a modest difference. If your push for dramatic improvement over short periods, you will be disappointed, suffer from burnout, and lose interest. Some people keep records of what they can do at each exercise session, such as ten minutes on the Stairmaster at a level of 3, eight sit-ups, and six arm curls with five-pound weights. This way you can measure your own progress. Some weight-bearing exercise is essential in helping to prevent osteoporosis. A good routine includes both exercising on your feet and exercising with weights, though not necessarily together."

AT THE beginning of week 5 I returned for my next scheduled appointment with Dr. Kass. After giving me an internal, the first since just before surgery, he was satisfied with how everything looked.

"The tissue is healing nicely," he said. "It's still freshly pink and some of the stitches have not yet dissolved, but you may resume all of your normal activities, including sex. No restrictions."

Those women who do go back to work are cautioned to adhere strictly to rest periods and abide by shorter hours. Discuss your needs with your employer. You may be able to arrange a modified work schedule until your strength returns.

I was dismissed and told to return in two months. I noticed a slight burning sensation immediately following the examination, but that lasted only about twenty-four hours.

The following morning I was back at the health club, where I spent nearly three hours. Besides swimming I also used the gym. I walked the track, but only half as far as normal so as not to overdo on the first workout. Most important, I felt, was to concentrate on those sagging stomach muscles. Sit-ups, done slowly and carefully, were surprisingly painless. Next, I permitted myself to push fifty pounds of weight on the Nautilus equipment, primarily using leg presses. By the end of the first session I felt stimulated, not tired or achy. I continued to monitor my progress.

Although this would have been the correct time to have resumed a normal working schedule, I chose not to go back to my former job because writing had become my priority. Those women who do go back to work are cautioned to adhere strictly to rest periods and abide by shorter hours. Discuss your needs with your employer. You may be able to arrange a modified work schedule until your strength returns.

Each morning I could scarcely wait to continue my research, as I pored through a wide assortment of books and journals. I read hundreds of case histories, each one quite different and unique, although I found a common thread. Every postsurgical patient experienced change—sometimes for the better, sometimes for the worse, but always there was a change. I could identify with these women because I was now part of their in-group or "club." I was also beginning to draw my own conclusions.

I had survived a hysterectomy without encountering any life-shattering experiences. I had lost my reproductive organs, but not my life. My self-image was strong, perhaps even stronger because I had assumed responsibility for myself rather than relying on others to make decisions for me. After reading and studying all available surgical procedures and their effect upon a woman's body, I was in a position to explore my options intelligently and weigh the pros and cons of experts in the field. Afterwards, I participated in the decision-making process as to which procedure best suited my own personal needs. My strengths: the ability to face reality, to educate myself, and then to accept life's changes.

CHAPTER EIGHT

SEXUALITY *and* EMOTIONALITY AFTER SURGERY

BEFORE MY own hysterectomy, I had been unable to speak openly about anything having to do with sex. Although any kind of self-disclosure can be both painful and beneficial, different people have different levels of tolerance for how much they can reveal.

In writing this book, I needed to relive my experience before I could accurately and sensitively deal with it on paper. It's neither an exaggeration nor a play on words to say that my life is now an open book. Yet after having undergone the surgery, very little remains private since the very nature of a hysterectomy involves a woman's most private parts, *my* most private parts. Despite my fears, however, I found that I had not lost my femininity, nor did I feel the loss of any qualities that make me feel uniquely feminine. I could still function as a woman and feel as sexy as ever—perhaps even sexier. The "new" me had now been liberated!

My own experience was positive even though prior to surgery I had suffered the usual dread of "female castration." Dianna, my coauthor and dear friend, questioned me further about this dread, particularly my use of the words *female castration.* (See Chapter 10 for more of Dianna's views about postsurgical sexuality.)

I informed Dianna that before surgery I had no prior experiences from which to draw to prepare myself. I only knew that my internal female reproductive organs were "at risk" and that I had tried to imagine the consequences of having all, or some, of those parts removed. The single thought occurred to me that the closest procedure to hysterectomy for a man was the removal of his testicles (i.e., castration). I even recalled this parallel being made in some of the material I had read during my research. The term *castration* struck an ominous chord, like I imagine it does for a man. This was the closest image I could fathom to capture my anxiety.

When a man is castrated, he loses his manhood by becoming impotent; even his "status" (in the world of men) is lost. A man without testicles, I imagined, would be full of shame and become the brunt of endless jokes and snickers. It was an easy jump for me to imagine an analogous fate for myself. My fear was that I would emerge from surgery a mere shell of a woman. With the very core of my femininity lost forever, I would never be a "complete woman" again. This was the beginning of my reevaluation of what it means to be a woman.

My fear was that I would emerge from surgery a mere shell of a woman. With the very core of my femininity lost forever, I would never be a "complete woman" again. This was the beginning of my reevaluation of what it means to be a woman.

Listening to these fears, Dianna cautioned me against thinking of myself as "castrated," that it was not a good mental image to use. Therefore, I caution you, too, about using this analogy. First, the very concept of castration conjures up so many negative associations, both physical and emotional, that alone can cause fear. Second, the idea of castration does not wholly capture the essence of what a woman experiences when she contemplates and undergoes a hysterectomy. Women are uniquely different from men in this aspect of life. The main difference is that removal of a woman's ovaries and uterus does not leave a woman sexually impotent or even sexually unresponsive.

The most essential factor to keep in mind is that your sex drive is a complex phenomenon affected by your brain—and *that* has not been removed! The sex drive is mediated by hormones that can easily be affected by your ability to relax. It is also affected by your beliefs and expectations and, most important, by your relationships—with yourself and with your significant other. We'll explore this point a bit later in this chapter. For now, simply remember that because the sex drive is so complex, each woman's experience of her sexuality, before and after surgery, is uniquely different.

PHYSICAL RESULTS OF SURGERY

Besides the psychological feeling of being castrated, some women notice a loss of physical sensation during sexual activity after losing their uterus. The uterus—that most unique part of the female anatomy—not only serves as a "cradle" but also plays a key role in orgasm. It is a powerfully strong muscle, and in its absence there is a definite loss of uterine contractions during sex. Some women remain unaffected by this loss, but others who realize the absence of this experience can be jolted by the harsh reality.

Unfortunately, physicians frequently avoid discussing sexual functioning. Yet the possibility of sexual dysfunction (either temporary or permanent) should be addressed by every woman facing a hysterectomy, and it is best if the topic is brought up prior to the surgery. Your physician has the ethical responsibility to inform you of all possibilities, both favorable and unfavorable, before any decision about surgery can be finalized. To conceal the possibility of sexual dysfunction, no matter how remotely the physician believes the likelihood to be, seems both unfair and unprofessional. If you experience sexual dysfunction after your hysterectomy, the issue should be treated sensitively, and your complaints should not be minimized. Your doctor should make every effort to determine the cause of the problem and provide adequate treatment.

THE IMPACT OF AN OVARIECTOMY

Later in this chapter we'll consider the psychological effects of having lost body parts. For now, let's focus on the physicality of surgery itself. One area of deep concern regards the all-too-frequent removal of a woman's ovaries during a "routine" hysterectomy. Unfortunately, many physicians still believe that any woman over forty does not need her ovaries anymore, especially if she doesn't want to bear children. This is an erroneous assumption that should not be indiscriminately adhered to by all women who fall into this category. Even doctors who prefer to remove the ovaries should raise the issue with their patients. Because each individual has to live with her decision, and because surgery is irreversible, it should remain every woman's choice to decide for herself.

What happens after the ovaries are removed? An ovariectomy unfortunately leaves many women feeling castrated. This feeling is real, due to abrupt changes in hormone production as a result of losing the ovaries, but the fears of "castration" may be misplaced, as we discussed earlier. The use of ERT replenishes a woman's natural supply of estrogen, thus relieving ovariectomized patients of the symptoms they would otherwise experience. Because removal of both ovaries causes "instant menopause," ERT can prevent the subsequent shock to a woman's system. However, ERT has its risks as well as problems. Proper dosage, whether in pill, patch, or cream form, must be adjusted to each woman's individual needs. This adjustment takes time, and sometimes failures occur. Those women unable to take ERT have no choice but to sweat out the symptoms of a "surgical menopause." Still, this does not have to rob a woman of her femininity.

Too many physicians are nonetheless quick to recommend a total hysterectomy with bilateral salpingo-ovariectomy, the removal of the uterus and cervix, both ovaries, plus the fallopian tubes. The argument in favor of this extreme form of surgery is that it prevents a second operation and is commonly referred to as "preventive medicine." The current medical trend is to remove a woman's ovaries if she's beyond age forty to forty-five. Some doctors even go as far as insensitively referring to this as "pelvic housecleaning" or "taking out the garbage." Many patients make the tragic, and irreversible, mistake of accepting this advice as if it were their only alternative.

The sole justification for removal of the ovaries is if they are diseased. Dr. Kass supports the theory that the only conditions that can be classified as "unconditionally justifiable" are the following: a malignancy, ovaries affected by endometriosis, or elongated fallopian tubes caused by a large uterine tumor.

Even if one ovary or a small portion of an ovary can be spared, it will save the woman from entering a premature menopause since whatever part remains should continue to function.

The Loss of Other Parts

In addition to the ovaries, the uterus is a highly significant organ and should not be thought of as just a "cradle." There's an old joke, first told to me by friends from South Africa on the eve of my surgery:

Question: Do you know the definition of a hysterectomy?

Answer: It's the removal of the cradle but not the playpen.

Nevertheless, the uterus not only is part of the reproductive system but also plays a functioning part in a woman's sexual life as well as the very essence of her virtual existence.

The uterus is a unique organ in the woman's anatomy. A powerful muscle, uterine contractions can sometimes be strongly felt during intercourse. Some women who had experienced deep uterine contractions and uterine orgasms feel cheated after losing their uterus. These are the women who report feeling shattered because of the loss of deep feelings of stimulation during lovemaking. Although sex is not the only component of a good relationship, it certainly can make or break one.

The cervix—namely, the lower part of the uterus—is usually removed during the procedure of a normal hysterectomy. A surprisingly high percentage of women don't know enough even to question their doctors on whether they should retain this part. Even after surgery I was surprised, if not alarmed, to discover how many women did not honestly know whether their cervix had been removed!

A woman might ask just why the cervix is automatically removed during a hysterectomy. The simplest answer is that removal of the cervix is an easier procedure because it is the lower portion of the uterus; separating it can be difficult for the surgeon.

Many doctors feel strongly about removing the cervix to prevent the possible occurrence of cervical cancer, which can be fatal. However, Dr. Kass indicated that cervical cancer tends to be a sexually transmitted form of cancer. According to *The Harvard Guide to Women's Health,* women of any age and ethnic group can develop cervical cancer, but African American women are more likely to die of it. Hispanic and Native American women also have a higher incidence of cervical cancer, as do women in Caribbean and Latin American countries. Lack of adequate health care is a probable cause for the discrepancy.

Risk factors for cervical cancer include multiple sex partners, early age of first sexual intercourse, a history of sexually transmitted diseases, and cigarette smoking. The human papilloma virus (HPV), which is sexually transmitted, can cause changes in the cells of the cervix as well as visible genital warts and has been linked to cervical cancer. In addition, infection with the human immunodeficiency virus (HIV), also sexually transmitted, increases the risk of abnormal cell development in the cervix (atypical cells or dysplasia) that can lead to a more aggressive form of cervical cancer.[1] Dianna points out, however, that proper use of condoms will reduce your risk of contracting HPV or HIV, and therefore cervical cancer.

Regular Pap smear tests at six-month intervals should be the only preventive measure necessary, although Dr. Sebastian Faro said that a Pap smear test does not detect HPV. Nevertheless, if an abnormality is discovered during a routine pelvic exam or Pap smear, it has been reported that cure rates are good when the disease is caught early.

The argument for retaining the cervix is that it is filled with nerve endings that can enhance a woman's sexual experience during intercourse. Yet many physicians fail to inform their patients of the possibility that pleasure may be diminished by its removal. Instead, they will tell them, unequivocally, that there will be no change whatsoever in their sex lives. It is therefore up to every woman to assume responsibility for herself by first being informed and then discussing the issue with her doctor since it is *her* sexual enjoyment that is in jeopardy.

THE LINK BETWEEN SEX AND EMOTIONS

Now let's explore how the mind-body link affects our sexuality. Generally speaking, a good sex life before surgery is a positive indication that sex will also be good afterward. Evidence suggests that women who reported satisfying and enjoyable relations before surgery were found to be enjoying their postoperative sex life as much, if not more. This satisfied group described their reactions in terms of good partner relationships as well as an improved personal sexual capacity. Women whose postsurgical sexual experience was less successful described the deterioration as the result of an absent, poor, or malfunctioning partner relationship.[2]

Because personal growth may also come from facing this life challenge, you may even become an emotionally stronger and more confident person. In turn, increased emotional strength and confidence can do wonders for a person's sex life. With these newly enhanced qualities, you may feel more comfortable asking for what you want in addition to saying no to what you don't want. You may also feel freer to explore areas of your sexuality that you had previously been too shy or hesitant to reveal.

What Is Libido?

In the context of this discussion of sex, an explanation about the sexual libido may be helpful. The word *libido* does not refer to a real thing. You cannot locate your libido in any one place in your body, nor can it be removed. The libido is a construct that was invented to describe the complex set of physical, sensory, emotional, and mental processes that interact to cause you to feel sexy. Some aspects of the libido are still not understood, but in general we can make the following points. On the physical level the libido is affected by your hormone levels, stimulation to your sexual parts, and stimulation to parts not usually thought of as sexual, such as the entire surface of your skin (e.g., a hug or cuddling may put you in a sexy mood). On the sensory level, how your partner looks, smells, and the tone and content of verbal messages can be a turn-on or a turn-off. On the emotional level, the quality of your relationship with your partner, your stress level, and your mood can affect your readiness to be sexual. Your libido is also influenced by your mental abilities to focus on your erotic sensations rather than intrusive thoughts that may interrupt your physical pleasure (e.g., thinking about the children, household chores, or a recent argument). So the libido is not simply located in a woman's erogenous zones; there is life after surgery.

> *Generally speaking, a good sex life before surgery is a positive indication that sex will also be good afterward.*

The Importance of Emotional Healing

Recovery includes both physical and emotional healing, and the two combine to affect your sex life, too. After your body has healed, it may be necessary to find ways to compensate for and adjust to any physical changes. Although scars eventually heal and become unnoticeable, that immediate feeling of lost femininity needs to be addressed. One way to counteract this temporarily damaged self-image may be by purchasing one or two glamorous articles of lingerie. Alluring lingerie translates into "sexy" for many people; treat yourself to something new if you're one of those women. Some women also report the need to find new ways of achieving sexual satisfaction with their partners; former positions may not be as pleasurable after a hysterectomy.

Dianna believes that emotional healing may be needed in some or all of the following areas:

1. Convalescing from the trauma of being physically cut in your most private bodily area
2. Grieving for losses that have occurred as a result of hysterectomy
3. Healing from disappointments that invariably happened when people close to us let us down at a time when their support was most needed
4. Being forced to come to grips with changes
5. Reevaluating the meaning and purpose of your life

Let's consider each of these aspects of emotional healing more closely in the following subsections.

Convalescing from Physical Trauma Convalescing from physical trauma varies from person to person to the degree that we, as individuals, are aware of our physical body. This difference is neither bad nor good, but it is something to keep in mind, particularly if you are the type of person who is keenly aware of your own body. I will call this type of person "body-based." This individual is more apt to become physically ill when feeling emotionally upset. She may also be more likely to experience an undefinable feeling of being traumatized and assaulted after surgery. It is important to remember that feelings of trauma and assault are the result of having been cut and physically injured (even though for a good cause).

Your body functions as a physical whole, so when parts have been removed, the body needs time to readjust to the loss. This is not just an emotional loss to which I am referring, but a traumatic loss. Your body cannot "think" in words. It can only sense that something akin to an injury has taken place. If you have this undefinable sense of uneasiness, it may be that you are a body-based person whose body is recovering from the physical trauma of having been cut and mutilated (from the body's perspective this was a bad thing to have occurred). Your body is geared toward survival;

it does not comprehend that it can be cut and mutilated for a good reason.

If you suspect that you may be experiencing what I have described here, it is important to realize that your body *will* adjust. You are not crazy just because you cannot make sense of these feelings on an intellectual level. Your body needs you to acknowledge that this was a traumatic episode, and be able to accept this period of recovery. Body-based pleasurable activities such as delicious, healthy, freshly prepared meals; massage therapy; nondemanding physical intimacy (being held or cuddled); pleasant fragrances; a nature outing or audiotapes of nature sounds—all of these suggestions can and will be helpful.

Grieving Your Loss It is a natural human tendency to want things to stay the same (or get better). However, it is nevertheless a fact that change is what life is all about. When life changes occur, we cannot help but think about how things were, and worry about what might happen next. Grief is about those things we have lost.

"I cannot predict what losses you may experience as the most egregious, resulting from your hysterectomy," says Dianna. "However, if you believe that you are grieving loss, take time to enumerate these losses on a sheet of paper. Next, spend time reminiscing about what you have lost, what it meant and what you enjoyed about this lost part of your life. Finally, follow these three steps: (1) state the loss, (2) understand its meaning, and (3) remember the good times. Do not rush through this process."

Tears are OK, too. Understand that there is a difference between healthy sadness and depressive wallowing. Grief is a unique process for each individual. I don't believe there is a proper (or limited) length of time for grief. Grief is only bad when you cease to take care of yourself or others. If that becomes the case, you should talk to a counselor, your doctor, or a trusted friend or relative. Grief can temporarily dampen your desire for everyday life activities; experiences that brought you joy in the past may feel empty now. Usually these feelings are temporary and your old feelings will return given some time. If your sexual interest is diminished or lost, you can use this time to deepen your relationships emotionally with those people you love. This can be a period of heightened emotional intimacy that may lead to more satisfying sex at a later time, once the grieving stage is over.

Healing Relationship Disappointments Although many of the people close to you will do their best to be supportive and caring during your convalescence, relationship disappointments are inevitable. This is especially likely following a stressful or life-threatening situation when most people's ability to deal with problems has been challenged by adversity. Stress not only creates problems within relationships, but also can magnify problems that already exist. Common misunderstandings can easily become inflamed. The only way to avoid relationship problems is to never to permit yourself to enter into a relationship in the first place—but who wants to do that?

You are born into at least one relationship, and that is with the person who cared for you as a child. Frequently that first caretaker's relationship can affect your expectations of relationships throughout your life. Are you easily disappointed in relationships? Do you end up in relationships with people whom you feel let you down? Even if you answered no to these questions, sooner or later you will probably be faced with a relationship disappointment. We all do. When this happens, you can take a few steps:

1. *Try to understand what was going on for the other person to cause them to behave in that (disappointing) way.* Ask questions to help you gain a better understanding of the other person's point of view. This inquiry is most effective when made in the spirit of wanting to understand.
2. *Clearly communicate your needs.* Sometimes a loved one does not know what you want or need, especially after surgery. Most people are eager to know how they can be of help to you. But no matter how eager a person is to be helpful, he or she cannot read your mind.

3. *Reevaluate your expectations of that person and, perhaps, of all your relationships.* Are your expectations too high? You can try to see that person as having many qualities, some of which are good and some not so good. You may even choose to keep a particular, though disappointing, relationship in your life if you are able to readjust your expectations and appreciate, and even enjoy, those other qualities that are good.

Coping with Forced Changes Being forced to make changes you may not want or like is a type of loss having a lot to do with your attitude toward control: how much control you believe you can have over your life and how accepting you are of change. Life consists of a series of changes; the only thing for certain is that things will change. It actually takes more energy to fight changes (because change is inevitable) than it does to make them. The problem is that most people do not change gracefully. They muddle through change feeling awkward and incompetent. It is this feeling of being "out of your element" that makes people try to avoid change.

We all struggle at one time or another during the process of change. Those people who appear to be changing gracefully are either more practiced at making changes, or just better at hiding their struggle. I am not suggesting that you hide your struggle but rather that you look at graceful changing as a skill that must be developed. It helps to talk to people who have gone through similar changes, as well as people whom you respect as particularly adaptable to and adept at change. Learn from them. This might be part of your mental preparation that we discussed earlier, in Chapter 4.

Reevaluating Your Life Any time you experience a major life event, either planned or unplanned, it causes you to reevaluate and sometimes reprioritize. The birth of a child, the death of a parent, a wedding, the loss of a job, a milestone birthday, a hysterectomy—all are events that may cause you to pause and reflect about what is important, and what is not. In this process you will likely need to let go of some ideas about yourself, what you had hoped to achieve or become in your lifetime. This letting go is usually accompanied by feelings of groundlessness or sadness. The feeling of groundlessness is due to having let go without having something else in place to hold onto; the sadness is about loss. Once you have accepted your new situation you may discover new freedom in choosing another meaningful activity. In the process of letting go, you may find enhanced appreciation for many things in your life as well as for those people whom you had previously taken for granted.

WOMEN'S COMMENTS ON SEXUALITY AFTER HYSTERECTOMY

According to the survey conducted as part of the material included in this book, two-thirds felt that their sex lives had not been altered by hysterectomy. We'll hear more details about their stories in Chapters 9 and 10. In general, those who found an improvement reported that their sex lives now ranged from "much better" to "fabulous." One woman observed that although her marital relations had gone through some ups and downs after surgery, now they were better than ever. Others emphasized a new freedom in being able to enjoy sex at any time of the month as well as no longer being concerned about birth control. (Remember, though, still to safeguard against sexually transmitted diseases by using condoms, if you are not in a monogamous relationship.) Many women, including me, noted the elimination of painful intercourse that had been caused by large and rapidly growing fibroid tumors.

On the negative side, one woman remarked that her sex life has never been the same since her surgery. "The desire is gone," she said flatly. A few others also indicated diminished interest, but even if their sexual relations occurred less frequently, most of them freely admitted that it continued to be a pleasurable experience. The biggest complaint of all seemed to be lack of lubrication (vaginal dryness). However, this problem would have been present in most women over forty-five regardless of whether they had a hysterectomy. As hormone levels decrease, vaginal dryness becomes more common. This problem can be treated in a number of ways, with ERT and/or vaginal lubricants. Those women who have elected to take ERT are rarely bothered by this problem. For women who cannot take estrogen replacement, the problem can still be easily compensated for by using proper lubricants. Several different types are available and can be purchased over the counter at any pharmacy. Only one person in our survey complained about deep penetration still causing pain even though her operation had been performed a few years ago. She also stated that she was having difficulty in achieving an orgasm.

A third group of women surveyed indicated that it was too soon to tell whether their sexual relations would be improved or hampered because they had not resumed sexual activity. Nevertheless, one woman said, "I very definitely feel the desire." Another reported, "We can't wait to make love. It's a major hormonal explosion. I feel very sensual, but at the same time have a sense of dread and fear of getting older and of having lost something of my youth."

In response to a question about marital difficulties since undergoing a hysterectomy, only three women admitted to having serious problems with their spouses or significant others. One divorcée said that she and her ex-husband had postponed a vacation because of her emergency surgery and that after she recovered he began to "hem and haw," delaying their departure still further until finally he left for a month's vacation by himself.

Someone else criticized her husband for being unresponsive and unsupportive, although she had described their relationship as "troubled" even before she had surgery. "I had a feeling of separation, but this—his lack of feeling at this most critical time—is what finally led to our ultimate divorce."

HANDLING STRESS FOR A BETTER SEX LIFE

The last woman's comments remind us that stress brings out the best and the worst in people, with consequences on your sex life.

"Good" stress can be energizing; "bad" stress is inhibiting, rendering it impossible for a person to get past a particular situation. For example, everyone's entitled to moments of irritability, such as PMS (premenstrual syndrome), a temporary condition. But when stress alters a person's character, this is a permanent condition and exemplifies bad stress. Stressful life events will magnify existing weaknesses in relationships, in a person's personality.

I experienced a good bit of stress myself throughout this process.

It was a jolt when I discovered my own need for surgery. First I panicked at the mere thought of major surgery, then I became even further agitated after the revelation sunk in and I was aware of the possible consequences.

Like many women, I couldn't speak freely about my concerns because of personal inhibitions. I worried, and even agonized, about the aftermath of such an operation. I couldn't accept even the remote possibility of being robbed of my womanhood. Although so many case histories that I read contained horror stories of "castrated" women, I remained determined despite these findings not to become part of their "sorority," if possible.

Although so many case histories that I read contained horror stories of "castrated" women, I remained determined despite these findings not to become part of their "sorority," if possible.

Prudence on the part of the patient cannot be overemphasized. Some women, like myself, are fortunate to have a gynecologist who is both sympathetic to the needs of his or her patient as well as judicious. Dr. Kass did not rush me into the OR at the first sign of fibroids; he waited to see what would develop. After monitoring my condition for more than three years and finding that it continued to progress, only then did he recommend surgery. Besides, he not only permitted me the space to wait but promised to try and save my ovaries if they were found to be healthy. Unfortunately, both ovaries had been affected by an advanced case of endometriosis and needed to be removed.

However, the ultimate responsibility remains unquestionably in the hands of each woman considering surgery. You must not feel intimidated about speaking out if you disagree with the advice you receive. If you do disagree, it is your responsibility to seek another opinion. Do some reading on the subject. Doctors are only human; they, too, make mistakes. It is old-fashioned to believe that you will automatically be well taken care of if only you cooperate, unquestionably, with your doctor. The reality is: it is your body going into surgery, your life being permanently altered, and therefore your responsibility to do everything within your power to ensure that everything goes right. Doing so will go a long way to ease the inevitable stress upcoming surgery brings with it.

A REAL TURN-ON: STRONG SELF-ESTEEM

A woman's self-esteem is very important, and feeling feminine and desirable helps enhance a positive self-image. If you feel attractive and desirable and sexy, you'll appear that way. It is therefore essential for all of us to maintain good grooming, trying to avoid letting ourselves become sloppy by ignoring our appearance.

Yet, good grooming is not the most essential element of a woman's being. The spiritual and intellectual sides of our personality come first. Good grooming only suggests that attention paid to hair, skin, nails, and personal attire is not just frivolous, but can further enhance a person's very self-image. You need not go overboard in this department—inner peace is more important than an expensive haircut or designer-made clothing.

A healthy self-image adds poise, which also attracts others. A discerning woman is aware of her effect on others; appearance is not just a veneer. Yet self-confidence is not born overnight but develops over time through a process of making decisions and taking action. A woman discovers more about herself as she matures—her strengths as well as her weaknesses. Because everyone has faults, because we are all human, it's the sensible individual who learns to accept these shortcomings and then compensates for them. Overcoming one's inadequacies breeds confidence and inner strength, which then translates into feeling capable.

Physical fitness is closely connected with a person's self-esteem, feelings of completeness, and it can also heighten a woman's feeling of sexuality. The woman who keeps herself physically fit by maintaining a regular exercise program not only looks better but also feels better.

Whatever routine you adopt—be it walking, swimming, biking, aerobics, even mountain climbing—your exercise regimen requires a commitment that you should try to adhere to. Inactivity produces lethargy, which creates flabbiness and unresponsive, sedentary people—"couch potatoes." Conversely, not only does physical fitness make you look and feel better, but recent studies have indicated that a person who leads a vigorous life will live longer while enjoying better health. It follows, then, that regular activity is beneficial for everyone but particularly for anyone recovering from surgery.

Besides your physical well-being, the importance of a healthy mental attitude cannot be minimized. Being able to turn off negative thought patterns or destructive behaviors and move onto a totally different activity is beneficial not only to the body but to the soul. The alternative, which translates into compulsive behavior or ruminative thoughts, can be unhealthy. It is equally important to know when to quit "doing," by putting a period at the end of a day to wind down from the daily activities. Saving time for meditation, visualization, relaxation, or prayer is also a beneficial daily activity.

My passion for books (both reading and writing) could be all-consuming, and intrusive if I permitted it to become a compulsive activity. Although it may be difficult to put down a good book or interrupt an exciting writing project, it is of paramount importance to remain diversified; moderation is the key.

Taking time out also helps redefine one's sexuality. Forget about cleaning that closet; the Sunday crossword puzzle can wait;

balancing the checking account can be finished an hour later; the car won't be repossessed if checks aren't sent out at that precise moment; even the office project can be completed after a break regardless of any possible deadline—get out and enjoy the day. A brief recess can take many forms: a leisurely walk (not a marathon), a bike outing for pleasure, a visit with a friend, a movie, a concert, a shopping spree, a picnic, a date with one's significant other. Whatever the pastime, it is healing. Dianna suggests that you will benefit from taking a short break approximately every 90 minutes.

The relaxed woman has a better and stronger self-image of her own womanhood. And enhanced self-esteem, in turn, will help you enjoy your sexuality as much—if not more—after surgery as before.

Part II

THE EXPERIENCES OF OTHER WOMEN

CHAPTER NINE

TWELVE WOMEN TALK ABOUT THEIR EXPERIENCES

THE WOMEN whom you will meet in this chapter were selected from the group who participated in this research, although their real names have not been used to protect their identities. They were chosen not only for the quality of their response to the questionnaire but also because they exemplify a range of attitudes and feelings of the seventy-five women who participated in our survey.

ANN IS an attractive fifty-year-old woman whose small frame and lively disposition belied her chronological age. A real estate agent, Ann had been released from the hospital for only three weeks when I interviewed her at her home. She had been referred by her doctor. She was dressed in jeans, and at first glance it was barely noticeable that she had recently been operated on. It was her slightly protruding stomach that gave indication of her condition. Ann greeted me warmly when I arrived at her home, and she welcomed me inside. Because her husband was away on a business trip, she appreciated the company. It soon became apparent what a lively personality and great sense of humor she had, but she also seemed restless. In addition, I observed how slowly and guardedly she moved about.

It had been nearly one year since Ann had complained of heavy bleeding and her doctor had tried to regulate her menstrual periods by placing her on HRT. Nevertheless, a week before Thanksgiving the bleeding increased and she began passing clots. It was then that her doctor urged her to consider surgery. Even though a few other possibilities still remained, the doctor cautioned her against waiting too long because he believed surgery was her only option. Ann's faith in her own doctor's judgment never wavered.

"Dr. Kass is very conservative," she told me, "which is why I didn't feel any need to go for another opinion."

Once the decision to proceed had been made, things happened so quickly that she hardly had time to worry. Just two days after Christmas Ann underwent a total hysterectomy; endometriosis was determined to have been the cause of her problems.

"There was just one bad day when I felt really depressed," she said. "I dreaded feeling a lack of femininity after surgery and the loss of my sexuality."

Nevertheless, to Ann's great surprise the fear of lost femininity was entirely unfounded. She revealed that she had felt utterly demoralized when her friend's husband tactlessly referred to her as "the hollow lady."

"Well, I don't hear anything rattling around so I guess everything's OK," she had replied to him. Ann not only felt younger after her surgery but also sexier and "clean!" she emphasized.

"I have a bikini scar, and it doesn't even bother me," she uttered jovially. "In fact, it looks like a smiling face."

Although it was still too early to determine whether surgery had affected Ann's sex life, she did admit to feeling "desirous" and hoped that her doctor would soon give her the go ahead to resume sexual relations.

She reported no marital difficulties since surgery but was worried about her husband's lack of understanding regarding the very nature of her condition.

"Not until after he had met with my doctor did he even begin to understand what I had been through and what the ramifications were for us," she said. Men frequently have misconceptions about hysterectomy.

When Ann arrived home from the hospital, her husband was out of town, but she was fortunate to have had the support of a grown daughter. Two weeks later her son returned home from college and was also available to help.

Both Ann's appetite and weight had declined slightly after surgery. She was very pleased about this unexpected outcome because weight had been a problem since her pregnancies. I was shocked to learn she had once topped two hundred pounds!

Besides her weight loss, Ann changed jobs. Her decision was prompted by her boss's insensitive and inappropriate remarks about having had her "plumbing" removed. For her, it was the straw that broke the camel's back. It made her feel personally unsuited for the job. Such callousness is usually born out of ignorance and fear, as opposed to malice. However, the effects of such remarks can make it far more difficult for a woman facing hysterectomy. If you or anyone you know has been treated in this way, it is important that you calmly inform the offender that his or her comments perpetuate an inaccurate and prejudicial stereotype. Also, you may add that such comments are inappropriate at any time, but are particularly improper in the workplace.

The week following surgery Ann reentered the hospital after experiencing pains in her groin, but was discharged six days later after the laboratory's report indicated a viral infection. Apparently Ann had been too active too soon following major surgery. "I tried to be superwoman," she told me.

BETH IS a warm, vivacious person who regularly attends a health club. I was surprised when she told me she was sixty years old since her slender build and unlined face made her look much younger.

Five years earlier Beth had undergone a vaginal hysterectomy, but not before consulting two other specialists after her own physician had discovered a condition called hyperplasia (an increase in the number of cells that can be the prelude to cancer). She also researched the subject, discussing it with other knowledgeable people before making a definite decision.

After the operation, Beth's husband and daughter helped her at home despite her feeling well enough to take care of herself. The only postsurgical change she noticed was a "loose stomach," describing the abdominal cavity as a "house without furniture." Her description of the empty womb struck me profoundly—the feeling of "barrenness" despite having grown children and not desiring more. Beth further explained how she felt that no amount of exercise would restore those slackened muscles, whereas it had been her understanding that vaginal surgery would avoid any discernible physical change.

"I cried a lot after the operation and felt depressed for several weeks. I got no moral support from my family, partly because they didn't know how to respond. The doctor had never spoken with them."

Her description of the empty womb struck me profoundly—the feeling of "barrenness" despite having grown children and not desiring more.

"What about the quality of your life now?" I asked. She paused a few moments, then responded.

"I take much less for granted. I think it has matured me and helped me realize the things I took for granted."

Although Beth insisted that her sex life had been unaffected by the surgery, she did admit that her ex-husband's unresponsiveness as well as his lack of emotional support was a disappointment. She had been aware of his inability to "be there" for her for some time, but his insensitivity and lack of compassion at this most critical time were what ultimately led to their divorce.

Recently Beth stopped taking estrogen (Estrace) because she felt it might have contributed to her slight weight gain. Her presurgical weight had somewhat increased, though she hesitated to blame that on the hysterectomy. She's had no complications from surgery and would "highly" recommend a vaginal hysterectomy as an option to other women.

CAROL PHONED one evening, shortly before the opening session of the workshop. A single woman of thirty-three, she had been compelled to undergo a hysterectomy four years earlier because of uterine cancer.

"But I do have my ovaries, so I won't go into a premature menopause," she told me convincingly, even though it did not negate the trauma of the experience itself.

Carol went for second and third opinions besides working with some excellent physicians who had fully cooperated with one another. Yet the tests had left her slightly debilitated because she had three D&C's plus two hysteroscopies within a five-month period. Nevertheless, she had mentally prepared herself for surgery by attending yoga classes, reading, and researching the surgical procedure.

"I read everything I could find, but there was so much negative information," she said sadly. "Even though I had no choice but to go ahead with surgery, it was difficult to hear about the awful decision I was making and all the problems I was likely to face. But, I still tried my best to focus on the positive." Carol also listened to audio cassettes on relaxation and how to prepare for surgery.

"I was very fortunate to have had my parents' help and support every step of the way," she continued, "as well as help from the rest of my family. But the help and support were not all that I'd hoped it would be. Even though they were there for me, I got the feeling that they would crumble if I did. I found myself actually helping them to deal with what *I* was going through. I needed to be the strong one.

"Being young and single compounded the issues I had to deal with. I felt I would have been better off if I had had a husband to lean on. I regretted being single more than ever. And, why me? I felt I was barely an adult.

"My insurance company wanted to send me to the American Cancer Society. But for me, a support group for single women deprived of their ability to conceive was far more important than a support group for cancer patients. Unfortunately, no such groups existed at that time."

Despite the seriousness of Carol's illness, she remained in good spirits after surgery by concentrating upon her recovery.

"Keeping a positive attitude and a sense of humor made the experience more manageable. But there is no easy way to cope with the loss of fertility. It is difficult even though I try to keep a positive attitude every single day. This was the real problem, the one with the greatest emotional impact. Although I went to see a private counselor, most of the time I spent educating *her* on the medical aspects of hysterectomy. She provided a sounding board, but I wish she had been better informed.

"My only positive information came from the HERS organization, which put me in contact with a wonderful woman from New York City. We spoke for hours. Although HERS had given me the names of a few other women to call, this woman from New York and I felt a special rapport. She was extremely supportive. Last year we finally met, and now we keep in touch to check up on each other."

Carol had carefully researched her options before accepting that her surgery and resulting loss of fertility were necessary to save her life.

Surgery had affected Carol's sex life. But even after confiding about its having made orgasm more difficult and deep penetration painful, she still found that most men did not shy away from her even after being told she could never bear children. At this time she was enjoying a relationship with a steady boyfriend whom she had already been dating for nine months.

Carol had also noticed some less stressful problems such as constipation, frequent urination, and the tendency to feel bloated. Though perky and petite, she acknowledged an increase in appetite and a weight gain of about ten pounds since the operation. Nevertheless, she would recommend surgery to others in her condition, but only after exploring every available option. Carol had carefully researched her options before accepting that her surgery and resulting loss of fertility were necessary to save her life.

SHORTLY BEFORE noon on the day of our first session, a woman emerged from the elevator appearing slightly unsteady while clutching the arm of a friend. I noticed her free hand seeming to gingerly support her stomach. As the two women approached my table, the one being helped inquired, "Is this where I register for the women's workshop?"

"Why, yes," I responded, but before I could motion her to a chair she continued in such a matter-of-fact tone of voice that I was startled.

"I've had surgery," said she, still standing.

"When?" I asked.

"Tuesday," said she. Still unbelieving I probed further.

"Which Tuesday?"

"Last Tuesday," came the startling response.

I didn't need to count on my fingers to realize that last Tuesday had been only six days earlier. Quickly, I invited her to sit down.

"What are you doing here?" I managed to ask.

"I would like to fill out a questionnaire and attend tonight's meeting," she calmly replied.

Gladys is a sixty-five-year-old who had just undergone a total hysterectomy because of a precancerous condition that had been detected from an endometrial biopsy. Yet in spite of her precancerous condition, Gladys's doctor had felt it unnecessary to make a vertical incision. She was grateful for the less noticeable bikini cut. Gladys had also received a second opinion from a pathologist.

Gladys had done nothing unusual to prepare for surgery because she felt that she had a very good mental attitude about the whole thing. Afterwards her family and many friends responded with help. Although it was too early to know whether or not she could detect any noticeable physical changes, at least she hadn't suffered so far from postsurgical depression. For more than ten years Gladys had been taking HRT and was continuing the therapy (an estrogen patch) without interruption.

She made it to the meeting that night, but I didn't know what had driven her to attend. Curiosity? The need for support? I hoped I would learn.

JANIS, at fifty-eight, had survived a hysterectomy for uterine cancer in December 1994, having undergone the standard surgical procedure customarily recommended for cancer patients. That was two years before our interview. At first she had been reticent about even filling out a questionnaire, not to mention attending the workshops. Nevertheless, she ended up doing both.

One month before the operation she had gone to her doctor for her regular six-month gynecological examination. It was at that time that her doctor first became suspicious of a possible carcinoma after reviewing the results of the Pap smear. She then had an endometrial biopsy taken, which confirmed the cell abnormality. However, before submitting to surgery she consulted a second doctor, an oncologist/gynecologist who affirmed her own doctor's findings. Both physicians recommended she not delay the operation any further.

Because of the urgency for immediate surgery, she had only ten days to prepare herself after receiving the second opinion. Yet she still worked half a day on the morning before surgery, not wanting to pamper herself but to receive moral support from her coworkers.

Janis had hoped for a vaginal hysterectomy so there would be no visible scarring, but her doctor informed her of its impossibility because of the presence of malignant cells.

"Not knowing just what to expect made me uneasy, but not until the actual morning of surgery did I feel 'emotionally dissolved.'

"After surgery I had felt a loss, an emptiness, because my uterus and ovaries had been removed. But the whole thing was still more like an out-of-body experience than a reality. I didn't become upset until after the doctor told me that 50 percent of the tumor had penetrated the uterine wall and there was also evidence of floating malignant cells. The scariest time was the waiting period for the results of the biopsy. That was a nightmare!"

Within a few days of the surgery the laboratory report came back with the recommendation that radiation treatment be started, although it wasn't mandatory. Janis was fearful of radiation and consulted other doctors as well as the American Cancer Society. A final decision against treatment was made after she had been informed that radiation could be more harmful than good by damaging healthy tissue.

Radiation therapy as a cancer treatment is able to kill cancerous cells by damaging the DNA (genetic material) within the cells. Unlike chemotherapy, radiation has little effect on cells beyond the target area. This treatment is not unlike a diagnostic X-ray, except for the time element. Radiation is usually performed five times a week and administered for several weeks. However, it does have side effects: inflammation of surrounding skin, swallowing difficulties, dry mouth, loss of appetite, fatigue, temporary hair loss, nausea, vomiting, and diarrhea. Occasionally, radiation can weaken bones, and there is even a small risk of causing another tumor in the same location. The degree of risks largely depends on the dosage of radiation.[1]

"Even my own doctor, an oncologist, told me he wouldn't insist that his own mother, sister, or wife have radiation, all things being equal." Janis opted instead to be treated with megadoses of progesterone. Progesterone treatment can slow the growth of cancerous endometrial cells in three of ten cases by counteracting the effect of estrogen. Estrogen normally stimulates the growth of these cells.[2]

When she returned home from the hospital, Janis enlisted the aid of a few close friends to help her through the immediate period of adjustment. Not only were these friends a source of comfort at this crucial time, but meals would have been a problem had they not stepped in to help. Whenever possible, her husband also tried to be of service.

Although Janis's strength returned relatively quickly, the long, ugly vertical scar had left a permanent reminder. Her body healed, but she was permanently scarred.

The operation had also put a strain on her marriage. Though she declined to provide the details, Janis admitted that the operation had affected her sex life.

She continued the progesterone treatment for the first five months before deciding to take herself off it. Even though her doctor had suggested she not stop treatment before the end of six months, she had been experiencing ill effects from it, including weight gain. After stopping the progesterone and discovering that both her appetite and weight had begun to stabilize, she opted in favor of a vaginal cream (Premarin) in lieu of hormonal treatment. Vaginal creams provide symptomatic relief, but only a small percentage of estrogen is actually absorbed into the blood levels of the body. In Janis's case, this form of treatment gave her relief while shielding her from side effects normally associated with hormones taken orally.

Would she recommend this type of surgery to others? "Only as a last resort!"

KAREN IS a forty-year-old woman who had vaginal laparoscopic surgery one year earlier. Her ovaries and tubes had been removed; her uterus remained intact. Surgery was performed as only a preventive measure because both her mother and maternal grandmother had died of uterine cancer. After consulting her own physician, she sought the advice of her mother's surgeon, and he then referred her to an oncologist.

Uterine cancer is extremely rare, responsible for fewer than three thousand deaths annually in the United States. On the other hand, ovarian cancer is known to be deadly.

Uterine cancer is extremely rare, responsible for fewer than three thousand deaths annually in the United States. On the other hand, ovarian cancer is known to be deadly. With a family history of cancer, it is understandable that Karen's doctor suggested the removal of that part of the reproductive system most susceptible to a carcinoma. Good arguments can be made for retaining the uterus, as we have already discussed, and it was not necessary to remove Karen's since her surgery was preventative; no disease was present.

Prior to Karen's surgery, when she and her husband approached the subject of her operation, she discovered that he shared her concerns. Both Karen and her husband had been troubled about no longer being able to ever conceive again despite the fact that they already had three healthy children. "I kept thinking, 'Who am I going to be after this surgery?' And my husband provided no reassurance. In fact, he was worrying about the same thing!"

Karen's homecoming from the hospital was made much easier because of the excellent support she had received from her husband. He not only helped out with the children but also pitched in with household chores and prepared the meals.

Everything seemed calm until her third night at home when, suddenly, she broke out into a cold sweat. She had a panic attack. By the following day she described herself as being a "basket case" because the attack the night before had wiped her out. Two weeks later she was finally on the mend, but not until another month had passed did she feel as if she had actually "straightened out."

LINDA, age forty-five, was a striking brunette with a willowy frame. She spoke forthrightly and without the slightest discomfort or hesitation. One wouldn't think she had a care in the world. Yet the much-higher-than-average incidence of cancer among her relatives was cause for concern. Four months earlier she had undergone a laparoscopically assisted vaginal hysterectomy as a precautionary measure. Two years before that Linda had a mastectomy after being diagnosed with breast cancer. Her mother, also a cancer patient, was suffering from a rare form of malignancy affecting the fallopian tubes.

When I asked Linda how she had prepared for this additional surgery, her response was simple.

"I looked forward to it!" she declared. "I went into menopause at forty-three because of chemotherapy. So a hysterectomy was not going to make much difference. I've had experience with surgery! I know what to expect and what to do postoperatively." Linda had been released from the hospital just twenty-four hours after the hysterectomy. Five days later she began taking long walks, and by three and a half weeks she was out jogging.

As to the quality of her life since the hysterectomy: "greatly improved. It was a relief." Sexually, Linda had already experienced the discomfort of vaginal dryness as the result of a chemotherapy-induced menopause. Now besides using lubricants, she also utilized a dilator. Although she is unable to take HRT because of breast cancer surgery being a contraindication for hormone therapy, she has done research on natural alternatives to HRT, such as Mexican yams, herbs, and soy. Linda is very athletic and remains in excellent shape.

MARY, age fifty, lost no time in phoning after being discharged from the hospital following a vaginal hysterectomy. Three weeks later we met at the opening session of the women's workshop.

A nurse by profession, Mary was well informed about her condition. She had had a uterine prolapse and knew that surgery was her only choice; restriction of activities and exercise had not been a viable option. Because her doctor had fully discussed all the facts with her, she had not felt the necessity of obtaining a second opinion. Yet despite her knowledge and physical good health at the onset of her first symptoms, Mary had, nonetheless, been mentally unprepared.

Her homecoming from the hospital had been simplified because her twenty-year-old daughter came home to assist her. Moreover, Mary's husband, a doctor, showed great empathy.

"I have great girl friends, besides," she added.

Nevertheless, extreme fatigue was something Mary had not anticipated. She couldn't believe that someone with her energy level could feel so depleted. At the time of our conversation she had not yet adjusted to the recovery process, because surgery had taken place just a few weeks earlier.

"I keep telling myself it's O.K. to sit down, but I also feel terribly sad." Sadness plagued Mary on and off for that entire first week following her surgery. For some people, activity is a way to fend off depression. When activity levels decrease, these people are more vulnerable to depression.

"I sat on my husband's lap and cried," she confided. "He was very sweet, and although clueless as to what was happening to have caused the onrush of tears, he was very supportive." There was a short silence before she continued. "I usually never cry or show much weakness around my family, so this episode was pretty weird."

When I questioned her about her quality of life since surgery, she answered, "I have learned to relax and have made big changes in my priorities. I work in my husband's office, but I feel a need for much more personal time together with him now. I feel like I just can't stress out any more, and I become upset over the constant demands placed on me not only by other people, but by myself too. When I focus on one thing at a time, it's better; I feel more patient with others."

In response to the question regarding her sex life, she sounded amused as she responded, "We can't wait to make love. It is a major hormonal explosion! I feel very sensual but at the same time have a sense of dread and the fear of getting older and having lost something of my youth." She paused. "My husband and I feel closer now than we have been in a long time. But I've been much more honest with him about what I need, what hurts, and what I no longer choose to handle.

"I had lost some weight before surgery, and a few pounds since. Now I'm as thin as I probably should be but have very little appetite. My doctor had already put me on hormones before this all happened—Estrace and Provera. Now I'm only taking Estrace.

"I wouldn't hesitate to recommend surgery to anyone who's having problems like I had. In a few weeks I know that I'll feel better physically as well as mentally. Probably, I'll feel stronger than I have in a long time."

A TRIM, fifty-year-old woman, Natalie had undergone a total hysterectomy in December 1993. She jokingly referred to it as her "PMS surgery." Prior to the operation she had experienced heavy bleeding. The one thing she felt her doctor had been vague about was what effect surgery might have upon her libido. However, she still chose not to seek another opinion.

Plenty of help awaited Natalie upon her homecoming from the hospital: immediate family, extended family, plus close personal friends. At the time she was unaware of any postsurgical depression, yet she referred to the quality of her life as being "almost" for the better.

Natalie and her husband's sex life went, admittedly, through some ups and downs, but "now it's better than ever," she affirmed. When asked to discuss any marital problems that might have resulted from surgery, she replied, "There were none that I hadn't experienced beforehand.

"My doctor referred to me as a 'textbook case' because everything came out 'clean as a whistle,'" said Natalie, smiling.

She talked about her initial weight gain, then how it had stabilized after her doctor adjusted the dosage of estrogen. She was taking a low dosage of Premarin.

"I'd never pressure anyone into unwanted surgery," she added.

THE YOUNGEST of my interviewees was Pat, who was only twenty-seven years old at the time of our meeting. Her surgery had taken place two years earlier.

Pat had been experiencing severe abdominal discomfort and had steadily been gaining weight when she phoned for an appointment with her doctor. After being examined, the doctor informed her that the cause of her problems was due to an abnormally large growth of fibroid tumors. Because of her age he recommended a myomectomy. This procedure removes only the tumor while leaving the uterus intact. A myomectomy is less frequently performed than a total hysterectomy because fibroids often grow back. The operation is primarily recommended for younger women who are still in their childbearing years.

Besides obtaining three other opinions before consenting to surgery, Pat read a lot of books and prayed. In addition to the comfort she received from her church, Pat relied upon her parents for help and support since she was very young and still single.

The combined weight of the unusually large fibroid mass totaled twenty-two pounds. A long vertical incision was made to remove the fibroids, but the aftermath of surgery had unfortunately left Pat devastated. The most disturbing aspect of Pat's situation was that it had left her permanently sterile. Damage to her reproductive system had apparently occurred as the result of the enormity of the mass of fibroids. For a young single woman who had looked forward to someday getting married and starting a family, the suddenness of her infertility had greatly destroyed her dreams.

The most disturbing aspect of Pat's situation was that it had left her permanently sterile. Damage to her reproductive system had apparently occurred as the result of the enormity of the mass of fibroids.

Pat began her recovery at home with the aid of her parents and best friend, but she soon became despondent and stopped eating. The very thought of never being able to bear children was more than she could tolerate. Her depression continued for two months, and she lost thirty-eight pounds. Only after Pat began to learn about GIFT (gamete intrafallopian transfer), IVF (in vitro fertilization), and ZIFT (zygote intra fallopian transfer)—the principal forms of "assisted reproduction"—did she begin to accept that all was not lost. All three involve the direct retrieval of eggs from a woman's ovary (see the glossary).

The success rates of assisted reproduction techniques have been reported to be as high as 80 percent. However, this positive outcome occurs only for those couples willing to take the time and pay the price. Each attempt to become pregnant through any one of these techniques can take a minimum of ten days and cost between $5,000 to $10,000, not to mention the emotional drain placed upon the participants.[3]

Because she had retained her uterus, Pat hoped that through in vitro insemination she could still become pregnant. She also knew that she had the option of someday adopting.

ONE EVENING, a few days after the workshop had begun, I received a phone call from a woman who was obviously distraught. Stephanie had undergone surgery one month earlier, the day of her fiftieth birthday. She had been experiencing very heavy bleeding for a couple days before going to the hospital emergency room.

"My doctor had told me to take three Advil, put my feet up, and lie down," she said.

By the next morning, Stephanie was so weak from having bled all night that she couldn't even stand up. Her boyfriend called an ambulance, and she was taken immediately to the hospital.

"By the time I arrived my blood pressure was so low that I was nearly in shock." However, she was treated and released.

On the following day Stephanie went for another opinion. The second doctor informed her that she had large fibroids and needed a hysterectomy.

"He told me there was no time to wait, and that he'd schedule surgery for that very Friday. When I reminded him that Friday was only two days away and that it was also my fiftieth birthday, he tried to delay it, offering me pills to stop the bleeding. Unfortunately, however, this treatment was only able to stop the bleeding for two days. At that point he insisted upon immediate action; the operation would be performed Friday, on my fiftieth birthday. He would not budge.

"Besides," complained Stephanie, "he had no bedside manner, and I had no time to think."

Stephanie believed that the second doctor had offered her no options, that surgery was a *fait accompli.*

Hastily she arranged for her boyfriend and children, a twenty-six-year-old son and a twenty-five-year-old daughter, to assist her at home after her return from the hospital.

"Before I knew what had happened, it was all over. I felt as if I had been railroaded into surgery before I could think and weigh my options. Then, when I saw the ugly vertical scar I was really upset and tried to cross-examine my doctor. 'Why had this happened to me?' I asked. I had taken an ultra sound exam before surgery so he had known the approximate size of the fibroid. My request: a bikini incision. His response: the decision would be made only at the time of surgery.

"After surgery, his only explanation for doing a vertical incision was that my fibroids had been too large to remove any other way. If I used the estrogen patch, he said, I'd be fine. That was that. Case dismissed."

Stephanie's agitation increased when her doctor allegedly became annoyed after her suggestion of possibly obtaining a book to read about hysterectomies. His response had been that she didn't need anything to read; she only needed to listen. Today many more doctors believe that a patient should participate in decisions regarding her care. A few doctors, however, still hold the old school beliefs that the doctor knows best and a good patient is a compliant patient.

Although Stephanie denied feeling depressed, she was obviously very bitter and upset. She had been unable to have control over her medical treatment. She had been a compliant patient. To make matters worse, her boyfriend deserted her, leaving for Palm Springs on a six-week vacation after she had planned to go with him to Mexico.

Even though Stephanie had not fully recuperated at the time of this interview, she had still gone back to work. She felt some residual discomfort, but the bleeding had at least subsided. Her hope was to connect with other women at the workshop who have been through similar situations and to seek help and advice from experts in the field.

TRACY IS a fifty-one-year-old woman who suffered from obesity. She had also recently been told that she was diabetic. She had originally registered for the workshop but then didn't come because she had heard it was for women who had had hysterectomies already. Hers was next month.

"I have heavy menstrual periods and I'm anemic. I'm trying to build up my blood count, but I'm worried about the diabetes—how it'll affect the surgery and whether or not it could cause complications."

Tracy's family doctor, an internist, had suggested the hysterectomy as a remedy to end her menstrual cycle because her bleeding was heavy and caused her to become anemic. He referred her back to her gynecologist for a second opinion. When Tracy's gynecologist confirmed her need for surgery, a date for the hysterectomy was set, and she began to concentrate on working out a diabetic diet.

At our last encounter, I learned that Tracy's surgery had been postponed until her diabetes was under control. Uncontrolled diabetes is deadly.

Mentally, Tracy felt prepared for the surgery. Her husband, whom she described as being very strong and supportive, had arranged to stay home with her after she's discharged from the hospital. "I've discussed everything with my husband," said Tracy. "We're best friends." However, she did admit to periodic bouts of sadness in anticipation of surgery even though she did not expect to encounter any major changes.

Tracy was managing multiple medical liabilities: anemia, her obesity, her diabetic condition, and a predisposition to heart disease.

Her biggest concern was gaining weight after surgery since she knew that women frequently gained weight after a hysterectomy. Although HRT could cause weight gain, she hoped her doctor would put her on hormones because the risk of heart disease after surgery is a major threat complicating her hysterectomy.

At our last encounter, I learned that Tracy's surgery had been postponed until her diabetes was under control. Uncontrolled diabetes is deadly.

CHAPTER TEN

THE WOMEN SPEAK OUT AGAIN

SIX MONTHS later, I interviewed the same group of women again, plus two others I'd met at the workshop, to learn how they were doing. Many interesting details came forth. Some had redefined old values, attempting to revitalize their lives. For others, new avenues were discovered—different ventures that offered fresh challenges and room to grow. Still others, more conservative in their ways, relied on old, familiar paths for comfort and continued stability.

ANN, SMILING cheerfully and dressed in jeans, arrived at this meeting with a noticeable limp. Barely nine months after her hysterectomy, Ann was facing additional surgery—hip replacement, and at fifty-one! Yet despite her ordeal, she still maintained a positive attitude with no trace of self-pity.

"My daughter's wedding is three weeks away, and I'm so excited," she exclaimed happily. "I have a beautiful dress, and I'm hoping for a dance with my husband. I'll leave my cane at home that night. Hip surgery I'll deal with later."

Ann said the hysterectomy had been "a piece of cake"; it was what followed that caused her so much anguish. Six weeks after surgery she began struggling with arthritis-related problems, which continued to plague her.

"I call this my lost year," said Ann sadly. "I'm just happy they have replacement parts for body damage so I can get on with my life."

Although she realizes that her hysterectomy was a no-choice decision, somehow she wonders whether it may have unleashed an otherwise dormant situation.

"My physical therapist suggested that the trauma of surgery might have pushed the arthritic problem over the edge. I knew I had arthritis in my knee, but it came as a complete shock that I also had it in my hip. Perhaps my being too physically active too soon after surgery was an issue, but I don't know. I was a bundle of energy and out driving the car just two weeks after surgery."

"Are you still working?" I asked.

"I'm on a leave of absence," replied Ann. "I need to wait and see how I'm feeling after everything's over. My husband has been great; he's very supportive. I am hoping to continue a productive life, whether I return to my former job or not. It might be fun getting back some creative pursuits, not only home projects but cooking and entertaining. That's something I haven't done since my children were small. It's possible that I will miss the challenge and mental stimulation of my job; I enjoy real estate, and I'm good at what I do. On the other hand, if I don't return to work, I'll have more time to travel with my husband."

"You look thin, Ann," I said, knowing how hard she had struggled with a weight problem.

"Yes," she admitted glowingly. "That's been a bonus! Some people I know have put on up to twenty pounds when they have a hysterectomy, yet I've lost weight. Perhaps all my nervous energy is keeping the excess pounds off," she grinned.

"What about your sexual life since surgery?" I questioned.

"There's been no change, actually," said Ann. "I do have some mechanical problems as a result of the arthritis," she chuckled, "but that has nothing to do with the hysterectomy. My husband's a doll. I credit him for my feeling so good about myself. He always makes me feel loved and beautiful and desirable.

"I remember asking my doctor if he'd permit me to resume sex, but there was a little red spot that hadn't quite healed. When he suggested I wait a little, I asked, 'How about having "gentle sex"?' 'OK,' he said, '"gentle sex,"' since it had already been several weeks."

BETH AND I sat together over a glass of wine, both of us appreciating the relaxation after a long day's work. She is a survivor, having risen above pain and tragedy—two failed marriages and two mentally handicapped children, now young women. Nevertheless, despite the blows she has received throughout her life, Beth seems surprisingly well adjusted.

"Life is not bad," she admitted. "I live in a condo, but when I retire I'd like to buy a small house. I miss my home and former way of life, but I get out a lot with my friends. We go to the theater and to concerts, and I enjoy singing and playing the piano in my spare time. My youngest daughter, who is twenty-three and healthy, is also a musician—a violinist. She's the offspring of my second husband and me, and the best thing to have emerged from that union. My older two daughters are from my first marriage."

Following Beth's hysterectomy seven years ago and subsequent divorce from her second husband, she "jumped into" an exciting new venture. Almost two years ago she just happened to be in the right place at the right time and now owns a thriving business. Beth sells health supplies—vitamins, herbs, and sports nutrition; she doesn't believe in artificial hormones.

She has traveled a long way since her surgery, that point in her life when she felt suddenly drained of youth, having entered menopause "overnight."

"Nobody knew what I was going through at that time because I kept it all inside," said Beth. "Had my husband been more loving and supportive, it might have been an easier transition. But our marriage was floundering then, and when I didn't get the support I needed from him, we just drifted apart. It was very hard because even my friends made light of my situation. They'd say things like, 'Aren't you glad you're through with your periods?' People thought I was overreacting when I'd laugh one moment and cry the next; they didn't realize it was partly a hormonal reaction."

"Did you find that your doctor was more empathetic since you went to a female surgeon?" I inquired.

"No," said Beth. "Both my own doctor and her associate were younger, premenopausal women in their midforties; neither one seemed to understand what I was going through. I couldn't share my marital problems with them, either, so I felt very much alone. Additionally, I felt I wasn't treated respectfully; my wishes weren't respected.

"I had hoped to remain awake during surgery since I dreaded the after effects of general anesthesia. I had a bad experience with it years ago when, after a hernia operation, I became violently ill. Even though I conveyed this information to my doctor, she waited until I was heavily sedated and on my way into the operating room before offering me a 'choice': 'You may have an epidural if you wish, but we'd prefer your having a general—it will be easier to operate if you're not awake.' But at that point I would have agreed to anything! Afterward, as I had feared, I was sick as a dog for the first twenty-four hours. But I'm glad I had the operation and that it's all over. It was a no-choice situation since I had been diagnosed with hyperplasia, a precancerous condition.

"Now I've entered into yet another stage of life. I can be an 'earth mother.' Since I have lived and experienced many things, I can now help others by offering comfort and understanding. You need to have lived through a lot before you can ultimately be awarded the status of nurturer. In this new stage of my life I feel like Mother Crow for whoever comes along and needs my help—I am there."

CAROL MET me after work; she was working in the nutritional division of a major pharmaceutical corporation, selling infant formula and products to hospital maternity wards, pediatric offices, and ob/gyn offices.

"It's hard," said Carol, "because as a part of my job I see pregnant women all the time. It was a challenge for me to get through each day when I was going through all those tests before my surgery four years ago. Here I was, just twenty-nine years old, and diagnosed with uterine cancer. Friends at work tried to be supportive, but I felt like a tape recorder, having to replay the news day after day in order to respond to their well-meaning questions.

"Then I would come face-to-face with pregnant women, and sometimes it really upset me. I met people who were ungrateful for what they had—mothers of twins and triplets who seemed unappreciative of their situation. If only they realized how fortunate they were to be carrying those babies! In between appointments, I cried. By the end of each day I had a throbbing headache.

"After three D&C's and two hysteroscopies within a five-month period, I felt drained. After the first procedure, I was talking with some nurses in the maternity ward when my doctor unexpectedly encountered us in the hallway. She told me that she had just sent the slides of the uterine polyp to Harvard University at Massachusetts General [Hospital] because the doctors here [in Chicago] were divided over my test results. This was a Wednesday, and she said to me, 'Why don't you come back next Tuesday, and bring your mother.' Right then and there I knew what she had suspected but couldn't tell me—cancer.

"When I checked into the hospital for surgery and was given the consent form, I wrote down a list of instructions: (1) bikini incision only—if necessary, a T incision; and (2) no removal of the ovaries unless you are 110 percent certain they're cancerous. In addition, I had arranged for an endocrinologist to be present at surgery in case the ovaries needed to be removed. At that point, he would have extracted my eggs and frozen them for later fertilization. Fortunately, the cancer had been contained in the uterus and my ovaries were spared.

"What kept me sane was the knowledge that I could someday have a child with the help of a surrogate. This I would do only with my own egg and a husband's sperm, which is a process called gestational surrogacy. The most reputable center for this procedure, the place where they have the best success, is in Beverly Hills, California. There they do major psychological counseling with both parties, the surrogate as well as the expectant parents."

"Carol," I said, completely fascinated, "who are the women who generally offer to become surrogates?"

"First, a woman must have given birth before so it is known that she can produce a normal, healthy baby. Then, although some women may do it for the money, others have more noble reasons for wanting to become surrogates. One woman, for example, had recently lost her grandmother and not only was suffering a sense of loss but was also experiencing, and perhaps for the first time, the fragility of life. She wanted to do something good for someone else; bringing a child into the world for another couple was the most significant act of human kindness."

As I watched Carol's expression and the determination radiating from within, I was amazed. Here was an intelligent young woman who had faced a difficult situation with courage and tenacity and had resolved to live life to the fullest.

As I watched Carol's expression and the determination radiating from within, I was amazed. Here was an intelligent young woman who had faced a difficult situation with courage and tenacity and had resolved to live life to the fullest. Although one path had been closed forever, she was determined to find another way.

"Infertility is very painful," continued Carol. "I have lots of expectant friends, but I can't participate in their conversations because I can't talk about pregnancy. I can't go to baby showers, either; it's too hard. Women who can't have children don't want to be told that they can always adopt, either. They know that, but it doesn't eliminate the hurt." Suddenly, Carol's eyes filled with tears.

"You know," she replied, a few moments later, "my close friend once said to me, 'I thought you were over that and had put it behind you.' Can you imagine anyone being so insensitive?" she asked, obviously still hurt.

"This has been a bad year for me," she said. "My grandfather died Thanksgiving day, and I made all the funeral arrangements. My family and I had been out of town when it happened. I needed to keep busy, so I took over for my mother. Then an uncle died, and shortly afterward another married aunt and uncle died within a few months of each other."

"What about your boyfriend, Carol? Do you still have the same one you had when we last spoke several months ago?"

"Yes, and very happily so," said Carol, emphatically. "We both have faced many challenges and have persevered. We're both survivors. Despite a few fundamental differences, I adore him. He's intelligent, energetic, and handsome, not to mention supportive and understanding—qualities I most admire. He's also very family oriented, which is important to me. Besides, it doesn't matter to him that I can't have kids. We have our problems, but they're relationship issues. I have always been cautious regarding my relations with men."

Whatever issues remained in Carol's life, as well as unforeseen problems in the future, I knew she'd find ways of coping. Her attitude had always been positive; not only was Carol a survivor, but she was pragmatic. She accepted her situation, knowing surgery was her one and only option, but she was well informed, assumed responsibility for herself, and remained self-empowered.

GLADYS, SEEMING poised and self-assured, arrived a few minutes early for her scheduled appointment.

"I'm flattered to be included in this group," said Gladys as I welcomed her inside, "but my situation was very uneventful."

"No, that's not true," I countered. "Anyone who can register, in person, for a meeting just six days after being operated on for major surgery has not had an ordinary experience."

As I led her into the den, I marveled over the youthful appearance of this sixty-five-year-old woman and the sprightly way she moved.

"What's your secret?" I asked, smiling broadly. "How could you have been so calm and cool immediately after surgery? I couldn't believe it when I saw you at the workshop that evening. You had just undergone a complete hysterectomy for a precancerous condition, and there you were!"

"I've learned that pain and discomfort are relative. In fact, I'm used to pain. You see, for the past forty years I've lived with migraine headaches that cause such pain and agony that I have spent a third of my life in bed. Headaches intrude upon my entire life—my social life, family life, as well as my career. I live in fear that if I overdo in any way, I'll get a headache. It's been my life's nightmare. Any other pain I can handle; it's nothing: root canal, hysterectomy—a breeze!"

"What type of work do you do?" I asked.

"I'm a speech pathologist," replied Gladys, "but now I'm semiretired."

"Gladys, all of us in some way have been changed as a result of the surgery. It's been a process, an adjustment, that each one of us has had to confront. Perhaps it wasn't the same for you, but did you feel any different because of the hysterectomy?"

"It wasn't a shock—you're right. I had gone through menopause years ago; like a blink, and it was gone! When I had felt the first flush coming on, I said to myself, 'Ahh, I think it's a hot flash. I'll count to thirty and it'll pass.' I had suffered from PMS, so I wasn't going to anguish over menopause. Yet, I now realize I did make a mistake by not sharing my feelings about it at the time.

"As an older woman, having a hysterectomy didn't change anything for me. I had already been taking HRT for ten years, and I'll probably take it forever—or until I enter the nursing home! I feel strongly about the use of estrogen, especially since I waited six years after menopause to start taking it, and by that time it may have been too late; I had already acquired vaginal atrophy."

Vaginal atrophy occurs in some postmenopausal women who don't resupply their body with estrogen after its natural supply is gone. The first symptom to appear is vaginal dryness. The walls of the vagina also change; they become thinner and lose their elasticity. When this happens, sexual intercourse becomes painful. Now the thinner, less resilient vagina can be traumatized during sexual activity, causing vaginal bleeding. Weakened vaginal muscles can also affect normal stimulation and orgasm.[1]

"Although the pathologist had thought that my having taken estrogen for ten years could have been responsible for the precancerous condition, for me it was still worth the risk because of the even greater threat of heart and bone disease for women not on estrogen. I've already lost two inches in height due to osteoporosis and have arthritis—that's enough.

"Yet, even with normal levels of estrogen in my body, I did experience psychological change at the time of my hysterectomy. Just before my surgery I had begun seeing a new gentleman friend who's three years younger than I. I also had a big birthday around that time, but I couldn't bring myself to tell him which birthday. Certainly I didn't want him to know I was sixty-five! Nevertheless, it was he who drove me to the hospital on the morning of my surgery, and at that point I decided to tell him the truth. Facing a hysterectomy had given me the necessary strength, and the impetus, to speak frankly. 'How old do you think I am?' I quizzed him. Then I was startled when he responded without a moment's hesitation, 'Sixty-five.'

"I had met this man at a very low time of my life, after having been dumped a few years earlier by my husband of thirty-eight years. My husband and I had been college sweethearts, but then he went through a belated midlife crisis and left me for another woman. This is a wound that will never heal.

"The new man in my life is a gentle person and a gentleman. He's here for me. When I was hospitalized, he visited me both day and night. Each time he said good-bye, I felt as if I were waiting for the other shoe to fall. My husband's abandonment had left me feeling insecure and unsure of myself. With him I couldn't be sick, and I couldn't cry; weakness was 'not permitted.'

"Later, when I expressed these thoughts to this new man, he couldn't imagine how I could have felt that way. Yet, my reactions were based solely on my past experience. I apologized, by confessing to have misjudged him.

"During this new phase of my life, I feel as if I am enjoying the best of both worlds. I live alone, which gives me space and room to breathe. On weekends and holidays when I want companionship, I have that, too. Although I enjoy my independence and newfound strength, it feels wonderfully feminine to get all dressed up for some man in your life.

"I healed quickly from surgery because my body is very resilient. I also had excellent hospital care and great doctors. That makes a big difference. In addition, I had a wonderful network of support: first, my three adult children who all insisted, 'We want to be there so don't deny us'; then my personal friends of fifty-five years; and finally, my work friends, who also remain close.

"The bottom line: I'm an older woman who's been through a lot of stuff and have survived. I didn't want to make a big fuss over this. The key factor for a speedy recovery: confidence in your doctor and good hospital care."

AT JANIS'S second meeting it was painfully clear that she was under great emotional stress. Although her hysterectomy had taken place three years before, something appeared to be very wrong.

"My doctor has said everything is fine, but it isn't," she stated with obvious remorse before dissolving into tears. "It's been three years, and I'm still suffering."

"What seems to be wrong?" I asked, hoping she would feel comfortable expressing her concerns.

"It's a sexual problem," she confessed. "Things have never been the same since my operation."

Janis, being a very private person, preferred not to go into graphic detail about the nature of her problem. However, she indicated that "it" had put a "kibosh" on the relationship with her husband.

"Intellectually, he understands the problem; mentally, he doesn't handle it very well—it's a big turnoff, I suppose. Yet I try not to dwell on the sexual part of our marriage," said Janis, as if trying to convince herself of its relative unimportance. "Sex should be natural and spontaneous, but when there's a problem, the spontaneity is gone, and it kills the passion."

"Janis," I ventured, treading carefully, "all of us who have had this surgery have had adjustments to make, but after the initial healing any lingering problem is usually a minor one. It's best to discuss this openly with your doctor. Most problems can be resolved."

"I listened to the other women speak at the workshop, but none of them seemed to be in the same situation I was in. Are others experiencing sexual dysfunction?"

"Yes, of course," I confirmed. "You had cancer, Janis, but the cancer has been cut out; you're alive and well. You indicated that you had had a total hysterectomy. Could it have been a radical?" Radical hysterectomy is the removal of the entire reproductive system, including a portion of the vagina.

"Why, I don't think so," she replied, her voice sounding troubled. "I always assumed that my doctor had performed a total hysterectomy, but now I wonder . . . ," her voice trailing off. A total hysterectomy is the removal of the uterus and cervix, but not the ovaries or fallopian tubes. Total hysterectomy with bilateral salpingo-ovariectomy entails removing the ovaries and fallopian tubes.

"Maybe it was a radical," she stated worriedly. "I just don't know. That would explain things, wouldn't it?" she questioned, as if just having seen the light. Yet, without actually knowing the nature of her sexual dysfunction, I found it difficult to respond.

"Perhaps," I admitted. "But regardless, Janis, even if you had the radical form of hysterectomy it is not the end of life," I emphasized. "There are remedies for every problem. Don't worry. You can get help."

Janis felt relieved. She admitted to having painful intercourse after surgery but would check with her doctor regarding practical solutions. We discussed vaginal creams as a possibility.

Quickly, we changed the subject. Janis's first grandchild, a baby boy, had just been born and what joy! Besides this happy addition to the family, she maintains a busy social calendar while keeping herself physically fit. At fifty-eight years old, she's a firm believer in daily exercise and thinks nothing of a fifty-mile jaunt on her bicycle.

"It's great," said she. "I love it!"

Even though her sex life has been altered, perhaps temporarily, Janis and her husband enjoy many pastimes together, such as opera, theater, art, and travel. She also works two days a week in the admissions office of a local college and attends courses at a university.

KAREN, very tall, athletically built, and poised, arrived for our meeting, and we sat together in the den.

"What intrigued me about you," I confessed, "was not only the quality of your questionnaire but also your background. I know that both your grandmother and your mother died of ovarian cancer and that your hysterectomy, at age forty-one, was preventive—there was no sign of disease. Nevertheless, your response to many of the questions was minimal. I knew there was more that had been left unsaid."

"My mother was diagnosed with ovarian cancer in June 1992 when I was four months pregnant with my third child. We were very close, and I stayed with her at the hospital during her confinement. It was a difficult time because her doctor was arrogant, uncaring, and had a no-nonsense type attitude. At the time my mother and I needed someone with empathy.

"Two years later, in September 1994, Mother died at the age of sixty-nine. Up until her last few months she remained very active, playing weekly tennis and golf. She had been an athlete, a real health nut, taking mega doses of daily vitamins and maintaining a macrobiotic diet. The diet consisted of lots of vegetables and rice, no dairy or meat products, and several glasses of water each day. She also supplemented her diet with beta carotene—foods high in antioxidants and widely accepted as a method of healing, which help to clean you out. We knew of cancer patients who had reportedly been cured by taking beta carotene along with the macrobiotic diet." Beta carotene is abundantly found in both yellow and orange vegetables such as acorn squash and carrots as well as dark green leafy vegetables.[2]

"It was hard to see my mother go, not only because it seemed so unfair for such a healthy person to die but because she was really the only member of my family I felt close to. She and my father were divorced twenty-five years ago; he remarried but she did not. I also have an older brother, but we're not that close, either, even though he and his family live in the same town I do."

"So, what made you decide to have surgery two years ago, Karen?"

"It took a while for me to make up my mind," she replied. "I had been scared about taking HRT since I was young and felt that I'd need to be on a hormone supplement for the rest of my life. If I began taking HRT, wouldn't my system depend on it? I questioned what the long-term effects to my body might be. Could it ultimately be harmful? I also questioned the short-term effects, how HRT might affect my husband as well as my marriage. Perhaps this sounds silly, but I'm not a believer in anything unnatural; even my three kids were all born at home with a midwife and doctor. I debated whether or not HRT might even affect my temperament.

"I found myself going from ultrasound to ultrasound, hoping to find answers while knowing all the while that I could not continue to live in a state of limbo.

"My first doctor had actually been opposed to my having a hysterectomy at the age of forty-one. He advised me to hang in there, that genetic early detection was around the corner. Yet I was afraid to wait.

"Next, I needed to decide whether I should go for the total hysterectomy or just have an oophorectomy. I did some reading, material given to me by the second doctor, which is when I discovered that the uterus is not just for reproduction but has other functions. When I learned the uterus was actually the strongest muscle in a woman's body and played an important part in the sex life of a woman, I made my decision to have the oophorectomy. By the time I decided, I was finally at peace.

"I also voted against the use of synthetic hormones and chose only to use the creams—progesterone and estriol. They're great. This way I'm not digesting anything into my body—it's all applied outside—and it works. No hot flashes! I did have hot flashes, which began on the third day after surgery, and at *only* forty-one years old! That was very scary. Hormonal creams put an end to the flushes, thank goodness."

"How are you doing now, Karen?" I inquired. "Any regrets?"

"It's nice not to deal with mood swings anymore, and I certainly don't mind not getting my period. That's really nice."

"Prior to having surgery you had questioned your identity as a woman. Do you feel any change from the presurgical Karen?"

"No change whatsoever," she replied. "I was a little surprised about that, frankly. If anything, I feel more of a change now than three years ago when surgery took place."

"Would you explain that, Karen?"

"I'm more in charge now—more independent, more assertive, definitely more even. I'm no longer threatened with ovarian cancer, but I am scared for my two young daughters. Sexually, I'm not less feminine, and in fact, if my husband were here, his comment would be that his pleasure has definitely been heightened since surgery—better sex. I feel less inhibited."

Karen works out at the health club six days a week, her only employment being raising three young and very active children. At the present time her life seems full, but she worries about her future. Will she be restless? What happens when her children grow up and she becomes an empty nester? Will she be able to return to work? Karen graduated from college with a physical education degree, so staying busy and active is important to her.

WHEN LINDA got in touch with me again, she was calling from her car.

"I'm in the middle of a divorce and am stressed out," said Linda. "I can't meet with you right now because of the trial and my having to be in court all the time."

At the time of her first interview, Linda had appeared carefree. She had spoken both frankly and with utmost self-confidence. I remember being surprised when she had mentioned, in a very matter-of-fact way, having undergone a mastectomy two years before her hysterectomy. Linda was also the one who had been discharged from the hospital just twenty-four hours after her surgery and by three and a half weeks was out jogging. Now her situation had radically changed.

"I understand," came my reply, not wanting her to feel unnecessary pressure. "I'm sorry to hear about this, Linda. I had hoped we might briefly get together, but now I understand why I had such a difficult time reaching you," I said, pausing momentarily to reflect.

"Could we possibly get together one evening?" I suggested. "I could meet you at your house, or you're welcome to come to my home."

"No," she replied. "My husband still lives at the house, which is difficult, and by the time I get home each night I'm too tired to leave and go anywhere. I'm really stressed."

The contrast between Linda's present tension and former calm left me concerned. She had had such a positive outlook on life, having undergone a hysterectomy at age forty-five. But she had no fear of surgery. She was an athlete and quickly bounced back. Now, however, I knew there was nothing I could do except to back off, which I did.

A BEAUTIFUL, perky blonde met me at the door for my next scheduled appointment. Mary had traded in her short, silver locks for something new. Barely five feet three, her youthful figure and latest hairdo made her appear more like a teenager than a fifty-one-year-old woman. Yet the new look was wonderful, not inappropriate.

"Mary!" I exclaimed, pausing only momentarily after not immediately recognizing her. "You changed your hair. You look great!"

Smiling broadly, Mary responded, "Yes, I did it several months ago. It was time for a change."

As I ushered her into the den, I marveled over the recent transformation. Since her surgery eight months ago for a uterine prolapse, Mary chose not to return to the pace of her former lifestyle. No longer did she feel the urgency to push herself to the edge. She was still assisting her husband, a vascular surgeon, as an office nurse but had hired extra help. Although it was hard for Mary to give up total control, she learned to delegate work to their two new part-timers.

"For years I had run on nervous energy, but as I began coming to grips with my own mortality, I realized I'd been too busy to really enjoy life. We live a block from the lake, yet I had seldom been down there since we moved into the house years ago. Now, I frequently take my three dogs out for a walk along the beach. You know, it's nice to stop and smell the roses.

"I'm no longer obsessed with exhausting seventy-minute exercise sessions three to four times a week, either. That was too much for me. I was obsessive about exercise; it became more of a priority than it should have. My exercise routine was unhealthy.

"At the same time, however, my husband has been busier than ever. Our son's wedding is in two weeks, and we're doing something unprecedented: taking nine days off! My husband's a workaholic, and he's worried about not having a practice by the time we get back to the office. I think he's suffering a midlife crisis; his fiftieth birthday is coming up, and he's panicked. He has become obsessed not only with his work but with his exercise routine as well. He's killing himself at work, and then killing himself to keep up his looks. He's doing what I used to do, but I'm reformed now!"

"How are you doing physically, Mary?" I inquired.

"I really feel very good—in fact, even better than before," she answered. "I'm more energetic, though I'm still as nervous as always."

"But you always seem so controlled," I commented.

"The more chaos in my life, the better I am at keeping things together," replied Mary. "But unfortunately I can totally lose it at times with the people whom I care about the most."

"Mary, how has the surgery affected your self-image?"

"I feel a loss," she said, pausing a moment as if to formulate her thinking carefully. "I've entered a new stage in my life; it's undeniable. After having a hysterectomy, I know I can never again be a mother, not that I *would* or *could* have at the age of fifty-one. Yet there's a difference between what you psychologically understand and the emotional aspect regarding the finality of one's loss of fertility after surgery. I had begun taking hormones very early, about five years ago, even though I was still getting my period. My estrogen level was low and I was going through perimenopause. After surgery, I continued the estrogen, but at least I was able to stop taking Provera [a synthetic form of progesterone]. So nothing really changed as far as taking hormones was concerned. Nevertheless, a hysterectomy clearly marks a new passage of life—there's a change."

> *"After having a hysterectomy, I know I can never again be a mother, not that I* would *or* could *have at the age of fifty-one. Yet there's a difference between what you psychologically understand and the emotional aspect regarding the finality of one's loss of fertility after surgery."*

"What about sex? Is everything the same, or have you noticed some change?"

"Sex is still great," she said, smiling. "It was terribly exciting for a while after surgery. Could it have been hormonal? Perhaps; I don't really know, but I was feeling really desirous then. Maybe I just needed to know that everything still worked. I think I was also concerned about my husband's reaction toward me after the hysterectomy. Would I be as sexually exciting to him? But I discovered no change in that part of my life. Everything still works and feels the same as before."

"In general, Mary, how would you evaluate your outlook on life now, postsurgically?"

"I'm taking my time with everything I do; my priorities have changed."

WHEN NATALIE returned for her second meeting, I couldn't help but recall the first time we had met. She had approached me at the health club on her way into the women's locker room. She had felt rushed and hassled then, knowing her husband would be impatiently waiting for her to join him.

Now as we sat quietly enjoying the solitude of my den, I reminded Natalie of our first session when her husband had become very angry over her filling out the questionnaire.

"He is very possessive," she replied, "and wants to be my central focus. It annoys him to see me going off without him."

This was Natalie's second marriage; her first, which had been childless, ended after just seven years. Natalie was thirty years old and well established in her career when she met her present husband. For over ten years she had worked in the field of marketing research, then switched to publishing and advertising after receiving her MBA.

Natalie's husband, age fifty-four and three years her senior, had been married before, too, and entered this second marriage with two children, a son and a daughter. Natalie stepped into an already established household as the somewhat infamous stepmother. She and her husband then had one child together, a son now seventeen years old and living away from home at an eastern boarding school.

"My hysterectomy was four years ago," said Natalie, "and that was a hectic time in my life. We had just celebrated our son's bar mitzvah, and before I knew what hit me, I was dealing with the aftermath of surgery. I had a huge fibroid uterine tumor that had been very uncomfortable, so I had no choice other than to undergo surgery.

"People told me that it would take six months to recover and that I shouldn't be distressed if I couldn't bounce right back. My husband could not believe the recuperation period might take that long. Yet it was a full six months before I regained my normal energy as well as my interest in doing things again. When my husband realized that I was finally getting back my old spunk, he exclaimed, 'Oh, no! Not all that energy again!'

> *My husband could not believe the recuperation period might take that long. Yet it was a full six months before I regained my normal energy as well as my interest in doing things again.*

"Psychologically, I wasn't badly affected by the surgery. I was forty-seven years old, through raising my kids, and I didn't want more babies. Also, I felt as if a major nuisance had been eliminated from my life: periods and PMS.

"However, doctors don't tell you that your sex drive may also be affected, and that came as quite a shock! For the first six to eight weeks following surgery my libido fluctuated wildly, but I couldn't do anything about it even when I wanted to. Afterward, when we could resume sex, my desire flattened out to zero. I had no interest, no response, and I was terrified—and angry that I hadn't been warned. Gradually, after my desire returned I knew that everything would be OK."

"How did having a hysterectomy affect your self-image?" I asked Natalie.

"Before the hysterectomy I hadn't thought much about menopause, although I had wondered if I'd feel older and less feminine when the time eventually came."

"And did you?" I asked.

"Never older, but I did feel sexless during that brief period when I seemed to have lost my libido."

"What about your relationship with your husband?" I continued. Natalie then became pensive. When she spoke, her mood seemed darker.

"My husband was very appropriately helpful and nurturing, but he would have reacted the same way had I been operated on for an appendectomy or anything else. The bikini scar is nearly invisible, and he has always been physically attracted to me as a woman. I don't think the hysterectomy had any impact on our relationship."

"How are things now?" I pursued.

"We're in a transition stage, frankly, and it won't surprise me a bit if my life stays as is or even changes dramatically."

"What do you mean, Natalie?" I inquired.

"We became empty nesters very suddenly," she continued, "after it was decided that our son should leave his public high school and enroll in boarding school. He had been unhappy with his life in the public school system. He's exceptionally bright, but he has struggled all his life with ADD [attention deficit disorder], and because of it, I gave up my full-time career to be home with him. That was scary, since working had been my life. Then, after being home with him all that time and being so close to him, I was mentally unprepared for his sudden departure. It was a shock.

"As empty nesters, my husband and I have now come face to face with both the strengths and weaknesses of our relationship. I'm hesitant to predict what the future may hold. We're both very intense people; I guess we must wait and see."

"How do you balance each other out?" I asked.

"That's a difficult one," she conceded. "The only things we really do together on a regular basis include eating, movies, and the theater. We also travel a lot, but that's not easy because it becomes a stressful event rather than something enjoyable."

"Are you happy, Natalie?" I asked, somewhat tentatively.

"I've always been happy; even when I was miserable, I was happy. To know I'm alive, to be really involved in things, to feel things strongly—this, to me, is what counts in life. To feel nothing—that is the worst!"

I GLANCED at the clock and realized that my 9:00 A.M. interview with Pat was almost thirty minutes late. Early that morning Pat had received an emergency call from her father requesting her help with a flooding basement. In her rush to leave for her father's house, she'd forgotten to phone me. Only after I reached her at work later that day did I learn why she hadn't come for the scheduled interview. We arranged a telephone conference instead.

Pat, the twenty-seven-year-old, was employed as an assistant office manager for a car dealership. When we had first met, she was also working part-time at a health club to earn extra money for college. Unfortunately, however, she left the health club job after she passed out one day while on duty. She quickly realized the difficulty of holding down two positions simultaneously because it had apparently exceeded her level of energy. Nevertheless, she finally achieved her goal by raising the necessary funds to enter college. Four months after this interview she was off and on her way—a university freshman in a four-year program to earn a bachelor of arts.

"How are you doing otherwise?" I asked.

"I'm feeling great," said she. "I went to the doctor a month ago, and the fibroids have not grown back. He said I'm OK. I'm so glad it's behind me.

"My second cousin just had the same operation three years ago, but her tumors weighed only ten pounds. [Pat's fibroids weighed twenty-two pounds, causing sterility.] It seems to run in my family, although my cousin and I were the only ones who needed surgery. My grandmother, my mother, and my sister have fibroids, too, but theirs are not so big. I've read a lot of books; they say fibroids are hereditary for African-American women, so I've changed my diet. I don't eat much red meat anymore, but I eat lots of vegetables, drink lots of water, and I've cut down on smoking."

"How's your social life?" I inquired.

"My boyfriend and I broke up, but I'm traveling a lot. I've been down south, to Florida, and I'm going to Jamaica soon with a group of girl friends.

"I still hope to have a baby someday, but I'm single now and I'm going to college soon. When I get married and can save some money, I know the GIFT and ZIFT programs can help me through the process of artificial insemination. But right now, I don't have a serious boyfriend."

I wished Pat good luck, and she promised to keep in touch.

NOT ONLY had Stephanie's anger toward her surgeon subsided, but she had made peace and was still under his gynecological care. She reported feeling pleased with the surgery overall.

"I feel so much better as a result of the hysterectomy," she admitted. As an advertising agent who sells time for a trade magazine, Stephanie leads a busy, active life. She is also sexually active.

"My first sexual experience after surgery was quite exceptional," she confided. "I was worried that surgery might ruin my ability to enjoy sex, but was I wrong! It was better than ever. I discovered that orgasms were as good, if not better, than before, and everything was rekindled between my boyfriend and me."

However, Stephanie had one regret: the "unsightly appearance" of her surgical scar.

"If it wasn't for the scar, I'd have no problem, but the scar is still as thick and fiery red as ever," she complained. "It's not even a straight line." She showed it to me; she hadn't exaggerated. It was every bit as red and visible as she claimed, extending from the navel all the way down.

"My first sexual experience after surgery was quite exceptional," she confided. "I was worried that surgery might ruin my ability to enjoy sex, but was I wrong!"

Because of Stephanie's unmarried status, the appearance of the scar caused her more pain and embarrassment than it might have had she been married. She imagined that each time she was intimate she would have to endure the humiliation of exposing her ugly abdomen. Without the safety of a secure relationship, she found this to be distressing. To make matters worse, her relationship with her current boyfriend seemed to be waning.

"He's sixty-four and is afraid of making a commitment," she said.

What I found most interesting about her relationship with this man was her ability to show compassion for his problems even though he had not always been supportive of hers. Not only had

Stephanie lived through a triple bypass with him, but he had also suffered from impotence that had required a penile implant. I was amazed by her candidness and her humor.

"It's great," she laughed. "He's always ready. You just pump it up and go!"

Eventually, however, his inability to make a commitment forced Stephanie to seek companionship elsewhere. She is presently involved in another relationship with a man just six months older than she, although he is not yet legally separated from his present wife.

"I informed him this summer that he must make a decision. He can't have us both, though he seems afraid to leave all the comforts and security of home. His home is like his security blanket. But still, I'm not interested in continuing a relationship with a married man. I told him I'd always be his friend, but that he had to choose: either his wife or me."

Even with this new man in Stephanie's life, their sexual relationship has its problems also. He, too, suffers from intermittent episodes of impotence, although it is not worrisome to Stephanie.

"Oral sex is wonderful," said she. "And afterward, his performance is good.

"I like to feel sexy," said Stephanie, "but let's face it: long, ugly scars are not very sexy! My doctor had told me not to worry, that nobody would see it. But that isn't true. As a sexually active woman, I know men do see it. I figure that if it continues to bother me, I have the option of having plastic surgery."

WHEN I next saw Tracy, she looked wonderful. Although still too heavy, she had lost fifteen pounds and was wearing an attractive jogging outfit.

"I never had the hysterectomy," said Tracy. "I went to a hematologist who put me on iron pills, and that corrected the anemia. I was also placed on hormones, Provera, which reduced the menstrual flow."

"When did you learn that you no longer required surgery?" I asked.

"Right before the scheduled surgery I returned to my gynecologist for a pre-op [preoperative] exam, and it was then that he changed his mind."

"You must have been thrilled," I remarked.

"Mostly, yes, but I had looked forward to getting rid of my monthly periods. I hate them and I figured that at age fifty-one, who needs them anymore? I certainly wasn't going to have more children, plus my husband had a vasectomy a number of years ago so the threat of pregnancy was no longer an issue. Besides, we love to travel a lot, and it seems like every time we plan a vacation I get my period. It's such a nuisance.

"However, I mostly worried about heart disease, since it runs in my family and I know there's a greater risk after a hysterectomy, especially as a diabetic. My father, also a diabetic, was thirty-six years old when he suffered his first heart attack; he died at fifty-five. He was not overweight and didn't smoke or drink. Four out of six of his siblings also had heart disease, and my fifty-seven-year-old brother has had a triple bypass and four angioplasty surgeries. I suppose I'm running an even greater risk with the weight I'm carrying. But at least I have less of a risk for a heart attack with my ovaries still intact."

Tracy also suffers from fibromyalgia, a disorder of the connective tissue that is four times more common in women than in men. It involves painful and stiff muscles, tendons, and ligaments, in addition to fatigue and sleep disturbances. Because she had suffered from some depression, she was prescribed some antidepressants, which also help her fibromyalgia by enabling her to sleep more deeply.

Although Tracy still misses being a school teacher, she manages to keep busy.

"My husband feels there's no need for me to return to work. He's a lawyer with a good income, and we don't need my paycheck. But still, I miss those children."

In addition to spending four mornings a week exercising at a health club, Tracy attends art classes, spends time with friends, and visits her eighty-seven-year-old mother once a week in a nursing home.

"It makes me so sad to see her," said Tracy. "She's confined to a wheelchair, and since her last stroke she sometimes forgets my name and has difficulty remembering her grandsons."

Tracy's outlook on life had greatly improved since our first meeting. She seemed to have moved on with her life, and she was much healthier than she had been six months earlier.

I WAS very interested to meet with Judy, who was the only member of the group who had not had a hysterectomy. Judy is tall, about five foot nine, with a large frame, very thick and wavy long blonde hair, and a rather tough exterior. She had participated in the workshop only because of her very strong feelings against the use of HRT/ERT.

"I know there's a strong connection between estrogen and breast and uterine cancer. Even Dr. Susan Love [a well-known physician and author on women's health] is espousing it now. I've read a lot, and there are a lot of doctors in my family and two deaths linking estrogen and cancer: my mother had breast cancer and my aunt (her younger sister) had uterine cancer. I get very angry when I hear so much positive support for hormone replacement therapy.

"I'm not afraid of 'castration,' and I'm not afraid of getting older, either. I accept the good and bad in life, and when the going gets tough, I tell myself it will be OK. Even if the news is terrible, I've conditioned myself to face it. I've raised two daughters alone after being divorced at age thirty-four. While raising them, I worked my way up the

Judy looks good—healthy and strong. Because she does not believe in using an estrogen supplement, she's given little thought to how she might have done had she taken ERT. Any changes she's observed have not been difficult for her, just a normal part of aging.

corporate ladder from a copy writer to creative arts director to provide a good home. I'm a survivor; I don't need a man around the house. I'm happy alone."

Judy looks good—healthy and strong. Because she does not believe in using an estrogen supplement, she's given little thought to how she might have done had she taken ERT. Any changes she's observed have not been difficult for her, just a normal part of aging.

MY FINAL meeting was with Trudy. She was smiling when I opened the door, after having just dropped off her two-and-a-half-year-old granddaughter at nursery school. So much had happened since our last meeting! This former empty nester now was sharing her home with a houseful of children and grandchildren.

"It's rather crowded," admitted Trudy, "with all of us living under the same roof, and sometimes they're disruptive. We really need a bigger house, but we never expected the children back after they both were married. At least we finished the basement, which gives us a little extra room.

"When our son-in-law became very ill, he, our daughter, and our granddaughter all moved in with my husband and me. We needed to help take care of our son-in-law so our daughter would not have to quit her job."

A year earlier Trudy's son-in-law had been diagnosed with melanoma, a deadly form of skin cancer, and within six months he was dead. It is their baby who Trudy carried as a surrogate mom after it had been determined that her daughter could not carry a pregnancy to term, even though she was still fertile. Her daughter not only had endometriosis, but the lining of her uterus was unusually thin.

Trudy had initially approached me at the health club to register for the workshop because she was troubled with vaginal bleeding as a result of her late-in-life pregnancy. She was afraid that her condition might only be correctable with surgery and wanted to learn more about hysterectomy. Nevertheless, she was only able to attend one meeting because she was overloaded with responsibility at home.

"How are you feeling now, Trudy?" I asked.

"Physically I'm doing very well, but it's been hard. I go day by day. Our younger daughter, who is twenty-nine years old, and her baby also moved in with us after she and her husband were separated. So, we now have both daughters back with their babies, but without their spouses."

"Tell me about your pregnancy, Trudy. Was it very difficult to be pregnant at fifty-something?"

"Not at all!" replied Trudy, emphatically. "This was my third pregnancy, and it was wonderful, even easier than the first two. In fact, I even kept a journal. I did this specifically to share with my granddaughter when she's older.

"I had become pregnant (with in-vitro fertilization) on the first try. As a deeply religious person, a Catholic, I felt surrounded by angels during my pregnancy. Everyone—family, friends, acquaintances from work—they all treated me beautifully and with tremendous respect. I felt content and at ease the entire time.

"Every night my husband and I talked to the baby to acquaint her with our voices. We also played her a tape that our daughter and son-in-law had made of their voices. The four of us became a team, participating together in Lamaze; our coach even came to the house because of the unusual set of circumstances. When the four of us practiced the breathing exercises together, it was very funny!

"When I went into labor, all four of us drove to the hospital together and remained together throughout labor, and then eight hours of natural childbirth. It was a 'family affair.' As soon as the baby was born, the nurse immediately handed her over to my daughter, the new mom. Our baby seemed to focus right on my daughter; after all, she was familiar with her voice! We call our baby the 'miracle baby' and refer to her always as our 'angel.' The entire experience was beautiful.

"I had a semiprivate room in the hospital (my daughter and myself), and we remained hospitalized together for two days. When a nurse would enter the room, the comment always was 'OK, who is the patient and who is the mom?' It was funny . . . the 'patient' felt great but not the 'mom'—*she* had back problems. We loved every minute of our shared experience, and so did the hospital staff. It was a first for them—not that I was a surrogate but a grandmother surrogate!"

"Why do you believe the pregnancy went so well?"

"I had prepared for an entire year," responded Trudy. "When I decided to become a surrogate, I had already gone through menopause and had not had a period for three months. The doctor put me on ERT to restart my periods, then took me off so I could get pregnant. I was on nothing during the pregnancy, then resumed ERT after the baby was born.

"I also watched my food intake—no chocolate, sugar, alcohol, or caffeine. I ate for the baby! In addition, I had a trainer who guided me in exercises to strengthen my back and stomach muscles even though she, at the time, didn't know she was preparing me to have a baby. I wanted to keep everything quiet, not so much for myself but for the child-to-be. Kids can be so cruel, you know. I wanted to protect my future grandchild from those nasty comments coming from the mouths of their playmates—'You came from your grandmother's tummy? Oh, no! How could you?'"

"And now, Trudy? What's happening at home? How is this new family coping without their husband? Their father? Your son-in-law?"

"My daughter has not gotten over the hurt. She's sad and even angry about having to raise a daughter on her own, and she's angry with her former husband—that he abandoned her. Unfortunately, she has been so busy over these past six months just trying to survive that she hasn't even had the chance to deal with his death. There has been no time to mourn."

"But she's young, Trudy—she's only thirty years old. She'll find happiness again, and she'll rebuild her life," I said, trying to be comforting.

"Yes," Trudy agreed. "That's true. In fact, she has already attended a wellness center for grief and support and has joined a singles program."

"What about the child? How is she responding to her father's absence?"

"This is the saddest part of all because she's too young to understand what happened to her daddy. Every day she asks for him, and when she does, we're honest. We hope she'll remember him, but we realize it's doubtful since she's so young. It's a pity."

"And you, Trudy? How are you dealing now?"

"Physically, very well. The bleeding of six months ago finally stopped after my doctor put me back on Premarin. Mentally, my life's in chaos. I have no time for myself. I'm an unselfish person, and that can be a curse in some ways, since I have a tendency to take on too much—more than I can comfortably handle. I don't know how to say no."

Looking at her now, I understood.

"There's a parallel here, Trudy. We've all been going through a difficult process this year, you included. The other women and I lost our ability to ever again bear children when we had our surgeries. On the other hand, you were blessed with a rare opportunity—being able, one last time, to bring new life into this world and give your daughter the gift she never would have had without you. Unfortunately, there was a trade-off, it seems, and you suffered a grievous loss with the death of your son-in-law. But, this difficult time will pass because the three of you have each other. You're a wonderful role model, Trudy."

When she left, I felt new inspiration. Trudy was a remarkable person—a gentle and loving wife, mother, and grandmother; somebody so unselfish as never to put her needs ahead of others. With her spirit, I knew their family unit would survive.

CHAPTER ELEVEN

YOUR OWN STORY

By now you have probably read my story, as well as the excerpts from my interviews with several other women. Yet these stories are not representative of all women or even most women. According to the *New York Times,* about 590,000 women in the United States undergo a hysterectomy every year. This rate is among the world's highest but appears to be decreasing as both doctors and patients reevaluate the need for hysterectomy and new treatments and procedures are devised. The stories included in this book cannot possibly capture the diversity of stories that remain untold. And the most important story of all has yet to be told: *your* story.

This chapter is devoted to you, the woman whose story is yet to be told. The goal of this chapter is to help you take a closer look at yourself—the main character—and the people who comprise your supporting cast (doctor, family, friends). The purpose of this closer look is to help you evaluate your present situation and to help you be well prepared.

No one knows what kind of struggles or challenge may lay ahead of you. However, I know that it is you who must put forth the most effort and take the greatest responsibility in facing those struggles and challenges. It is also you who are in the best position to know just what resources you can rely on and what things might possibly undermine you during this difficult challenge ahead. Self-awareness is the means to this understanding.

Self-awareness, knowing what causes you stress and what brings you comfort, can be very valuable throughout life but particularly as you prepare for major surgery such as a hysterectomy. If you know what kinds of situations or people stress you out, you can prepare yourself or even improve yourself so you can handle those things most effectively. Generally, people experience less stress and feel more at ease if they actively participate in their medical care decisions. However, the task of educating yourself, evaluating your options, making decisions, and taking action can be stressful in itself. Your personality and style of coping determine to what extent you are able to succeed at each of these tasks. The more overwhelming the task feels to you, the more you will need to rely on your social supports to get you through it.

I instinctively knew that being uninformed about my medical care resulted in feeling out of control, causing me stress. It was my natural coping style to take charge of the situation by learning as much as I could and being as involved as I could be. But you may have a different style and different ways of feeling prepared for your particular situation. Reading this book is one step in that preparation, but another important step in your preparation is identifying the details of your unique situation that are likely to contribute to your stress. For one woman it may be money problems due to lack of employment during the recovery period or fear of job loss. For another woman it may be caring for her children. Try to anticipate what will cause you stress and what will be of help to you. Gather information and seek solutions accordingly.

Self-awareness, knowing what causes you stress and what brings you comfort, can be very valuable throughout life but particularly as you prepare for major surgery such as a hysterectomy.

After acquiring information, the next step is making decisions. Some people move more slowly than others in making decision; they never feel like they have enough information so they just keep postponing. Other people avoid making decisions because they are in denial. Making decisions is a skill. The more decisions you make (or are forced to make), the better you will get at that skill. Most women are not given the choice as to whether they should have a hysterectomy. More likely, they are only given the option of when to have the operation. However, the "when" question can distract you from the decision of whether you should have a hysterectomy. Even if your doctor says you must have a hysterectomy, that is only one opinion. A New York physician, Dr. Stanley West, has taken a radical stance on hysterectomies. He believes that the vast majority (500,000 of the nearly 600,000 yearly) are unnecessary. Could your hysterectomy be unnecessary?[1]

If you are fortunate enough to be facing a necessary but nonemergency hysterectomy, use that time to prepare your mind, your body, your finances, and your household. Many of these issues have already been covered earlier in the book, but we'll review them from a slightly different angle here. I also will provide a checklist at the end of this chapter to remind you of the areas where preparation is recommended.

PREPARING YOUR MIND

Besides educating yourself, mental preparation involves acceptance of the fact that you need surgery (if hysterectomy is necessary) and acknowledging your choice to have a hysterectomy (whether it is optional or necessary). If you fail to acknowledge your choices, you leave yourself open to feeling like a victim, which could lead to bitterness and even depression. You must accept the situation, and then after that you must deal with the fears and concerns that you have about the surgery.

The best advice about acceptance is that it has to do with issues of boundaries and control. If you are a woman who has received the news that you might need or must have pelvic surgery, you feel your life is forever changed, and the realization of that change has happened in an instant. All of this happened outside your control. The reason you have been advised to have surgery also is beyond your control (e.g., cancer, fibroid tumors, endometriosis). But what you do as a result of learning is not out of your control but well within your grasp. It is important to have a clear distinction between what is within your control and what is not.

Another important boundary and control issue concerns your physical body. No one has a right to touch, let alone cut, your body without your permission. You have the right and the responsibility to control what is done to your body. This may be obvious to some women but not to others, particularly those women with a history of physical or sexual abuse who suffered body-boundary violations in the past.

An example of an attempt to control that which you cannot is trying to find an answer to the question "Why me? Why do I need to have a hysterectomy?" Most people ask this question as part of the grieving process, but they do not become fixated on it. This question seldom has a definitive answer; it is an existential question, the answer to which is based on how you attribute meaning to events that are essentially unexplainable. If you persist at trying to answer this question, it may be your way of avoiding action. Pondering "why?" gives the illusion of doing something meaningful, while actually you accomplish very little.

Something you can control is your attitude about the surgery and its outcome. Research has shown that people who have a positive attitude about their surgery or illness do far better than those who do not have a positive attitude. Some of these "positive attitude people" were reported to have a ridiculously, unrealistically positive attitude about their illness (usually cancer). Nevertheless, these people did much better and lived far longer than predicted (in the case of cancer) than those people who were more realistic. Apparently the positive mental attitude assists the body in healing in a way that scientists are yet to understand. You cannot be too positive about your recovery!

PREPARING YOUR BODY

Physical preparation has to do with taking good care of yourself prior to the surgery, eating well, exercising moderately, and getting enough rest. The surgery will take its toll on your body, but to what degree will be, in part, dependent on your physical condition before the surgery. If you are run-down before surgery, your recovery period will be longer and the likelihood of complications greater. If you are too busy or overwhelmed to make major changes, a few minor ones will still yield positive results. Try something as simple as eliminating fried foods, eating an apple every day, taking a daily walk, or napping every afternoon. You can probably find time to do one positive thing for your body.

PREPARING THE HOUSEHOLD

There are two ways to think about your household: the regular chores that must get done (cooking, cleaning, etc.) and the people who comprise your household.

You must plan ahead for your daily living needs, especially during the first weeks following the surgery. For example, I had all the meals made and frozen and had a plan ready to put into action regarding what I would do after I arrived home. Ideally these preparations should emphasize "creature comforts," but you cannot attend to comfort until you know how you will attend to the basics, such as having enough food and getting to the bathroom. When you return home from surgery, you will have been through a trying time. You will do best in an environment that nurtures you and allows you plenty of time to rest. Use your answers to the checklist on page 171 to help you identify activities that would be beneficial to you during this time. You may have to modify some of these activities because of your temporarily lower energy level.

As part of your supporting cast, your family can be both a blessing and sometimes a burden. Most women still hold to the belief that it is their responsibility to manage the household. If you have been doing this all along, other family members may automatically expect you to continue to manage the household even if you have just had surgery. Usually these expectations are subtly expressed.

For example, it is unlikely that you will be expected to keep the house clean. However, you may be asked seemingly trivial questions, such as "Honey, where are my striped socks?" Usually when family members seek you out in this way, either they are behaving out of habit or they need to make contact with you to obtain reassurance that you are OK. It is best to deal with these minor demands on your temporarily limited energy on a case-by-case basis. However, I encourage you to communicate your wishes clearly and gently if you feel the demands being made of you are inappropriate or hindering your recovery.

Some women feel guilty when they take care of themselves in preference to taking care of others. Putting your needs first can be difficult, particularly if you are not accustomed to that. However, taking good care of yourself is not only perfectly OK but the right thing to do. If you need to justify temporarily by putting your needs above those of others, tell yourself, and others, that the better you take care of yourself during your period of recovery, the sooner you will be fully available for those you love.

Other sources of comfort (or stress) come from relationships with medical professionals, relatives, and friends. First, remember that doctors are people, too. They have good days and bad. They are well trained and capable, but they are also mortal. It is extremely important, however, that you have confidence in your doctor, that she or he makes you feel she is trustworthy and will honor your wishes whenever possible. This is important because once you are anesthetized you will not be able to indicate your wishes (e.g., "Do not take my ovaries"). So you must feel you can talk to your doctor—at length, if needed—and she or he will listen. If you have concerns about your doctor's willingness to listen to you, discuss them. It is often the

> *As part of your supporting cast, your family can be both a blessing and sometimes a burden.*

case that the doctor does not realize how you feel and will be grateful for the feedback. Doctors are trained to work with the body, but your collaboration may be needed for her or him to understand how your physical state may be affecting your emotions.

Your relationship to other helping professionals, such as the surgeon (who may be someone other than your own attending physician), the anesthesiologist, the residents, and the nurses, may or may not be as important to you. You have a right to meet and talk to those people who will be present at the time of your surgery. Unfortunately, even though this is your right, it may not be possible under every circumstance. On the other hand, if this is your wish, you may be pleasantly surprised.

The other players in your supporting cast are your friends and relatives. They can provide valuable emotional support, encouragement, and assistance, or they may disappoint you by their failure to empathize fully with what you are going through. I do not think it is possible to really imagine what it is like to undergo a hysterectomy unless you have gone through it yourself. Even then, everyone's experience is slightly different.

Your friends and loved ones may imagine all kinds of frightening or disturbing consequences (just like you probably have) as a result of the surgery. Others realize that they cannot grasp what you are going through and feel inadequate. Most people experience some inadequacy regarding what to say or to do to be supportive. Others have fears about their own mortality and become overwhelmed at the prospect of major surgery or illness, even if it's not their own. They avoid you to avoid their own anxiety.

Your hysterectomy has a ripple effect, like a stone dropped into a calm pond. It affects you at the center and all those around you in both good and bad ways. Some relationships will grow stronger. Others will be shaken. However, the most profound effect will be felt by you.

All of us live our daily lives with a certain amount of denial about death. Although death crosses most people's minds from time to time, mostly we deny our mortality and worry about daily problems instead—it's easier. When you anticipate your major surgery, it is expectable to think about death. These thoughts are realistic. They only become morbid if you dwell on death and lose sight of life.

When you are forced to think about your own mortality, you have an opportunity to reevaluate what is important to you and, as a result, change your priorities. As a result of the hysterectomy, you will be presented with the opportunity to take greater responsibility for your own well-being, appreciate life more completely, and love more fully.

NURTURING ACTIVITIES SUITABLE FOR YOUR RECOVERY

- Walking
- Watching movies
- Reading
- Socializing (in person, via telephone, on the Internet)
- Writing (letters, a journal, creative writing)
- Relaxing
- Meditating
- Praying
- Listening to or playing music
- Drawing and painting
- Doing crafts
- Napping
- Eating chocolate (in moderation)
- Eating ice cream (in moderation)
- Massaging
- Getting a massage
- Working puzzles

- Playing board or card games
- Listening to audiotape programs

YOUR PREPARATION CHECKLIST

1. Do you have these valuable skills?
    - Assertiveness
    - Problem solving
    - Goal setting
    - Organization
    - Stress management
2. Do you have these positive mental abilities?
    - Making decisions
    - Letting go of what you cannot change
    - Maintaining a positive mental attitude
    - Seeing humor in everyday life
    - Being self-aware
3. Do you have these negative emotional tendencies?
    - Worry
    - Guilt
    - Avoidance
    - Anger
    - Excessiveness in any area of your life
4. Are your environmental supports in place?
    - Household help
    - Bill paying
    - Food purchases
    - Food preparation

- Child care
- Cash available

5. Are you physically ready?
    - Exercising regularly
    - Following proper diet and nutrition
    - Taking medical advice
    - Enjoying proper rest
6. What are your social supports?
    - Family
    - Friends
    - Spouse/significant other
    - Support group
    - Spiritual community

Part III

THE SURVEY AND WORKSHOP

CHAPTER TWELVE

FROM CHALLENGE *to* PEACE THROUGH *a* POSITIVE MENTAL ATTITUDE

If my forties were a time of great excitement and turbulence, my fifties have begun more peacefully—a time of tranquility but also a time of change. Not only have I experienced growth and maturity, but I am in tune with myself, my new goals, my lifestyle, and even my sexuality. I know who I am and feel comfortable. While proud of my achievements, I'm also accepting of my failures. Life isn't all black or white but a symphony of many shades and nuances. Facing reality is the final acceptance that in all aspects of life both positives and negatives exist. Each of us makes choices. Sometimes we choose wisely, sometimes not; yet we must live with these decisions, and how we live with these decisions can make all the difference.

I had made the decision to proceed with surgery, knowing it was necessary though irreversible. I have no regrets because I not only had faith in my doctor and accepted his professional judgment but also had been fully informed and, as a result, prepared. I was thorough in my research. My body has been altered, but it's all internal; the physical changes are comparatively minor. Even the initial psychological shock from the trauma of surgery has since abated. Regardless of the horror stories out there regarding hysterectomies, it was not devastating. This does not mean to imply that all hysterectomized women have dreadful stories to relate; some positive accounts do exist. Life, for me, has not ended; only my childbearing years have come to a close.

Although the finality of never again being able to have another baby may seem like a loss to some people, to others it's unimportant, even a blessing. How you, as a woman, deal with the situation will depend on many factors: age, marital status, and whether childbearing is a goal of yours.

How you, as a woman, deal with the situation will depend on many factors: age, marital status, and whether childbearing is a goal of yours.

As a psychotherapist, Dianna encouraged me to understand how differently people view private matters. Each operation is different (some more extensive than others), but any form of hysterectomy is a serious consideration for most women to contemplate.

For me, that new beginning arrived after I had accepted the surgical change to my being. Realizing it was not a monumental loss but merely an internal bodily change that would have little bearing on my future life, I found peace. I discovered that not only was I the same on the outside, but I also felt little difference on the inside. Yet, there was a change.

Physically, I felt fine and resumed all aspects of a normal life. But personally I had grown and my life took on new meaning.

I recognized that my closest ally, most steadfast friend, companion, and lover was someone very dear, someone who had stood by me through thick and thin even when I, on occasion, failed him. This most special person, my husband Marty, is the one to whom I owe my deepest gratitude. His incredible strength, wisdom, unfailing love, and compassion were qualities that I had not counted on. This is what I value most, and I will treasure him for the rest of my life.

HAVING ARRIVED at this new place, at the site where I found peace, I began to rearrange my life's priorities. It was at this time when I found the desire and the need to help other women who were struggling through their own difficult ordeals. This is when my own hurt led me to the next stage: questionnaires and personal interviews of women who had faced the same life challenge. It was time to learn, firsthand, how other women felt about hysterectomy and then explore the issues further.

The purpose of the questionnaires and interviews was to acquire new data, and it targeted not only those women who had undergone hysterectomies but also those facing the procedure or who had problems that might someday result in surgery. Over one hundred interviews were conducted. In addition, hundreds of questionnaires were mailed to women throughout the Chicagoland area, primarily the northern suburbs.

Within the first three months, seventy-five questionnaires had been tabulated. Although many more were returned, only reasonably complete questionnaires were used for our research. The women surveyed were predominantly Caucasian, well educated, and middle and upper-middle class. Because most of them lived along Chicago's North Shore, the results obtained were more likely to be representative of people with similar characteristics. However, the study included women of a wide range of ages, from twenty-six to eighty-two, with a median age of fifty-five.

Of those women polled, fifty-six indicated that surgery had been required, fifteen said theirs was elective, and four abstained from answering. Of the women who required hysterectomies, six reported malignancies, whereas eight had precancerous conditions.

One of the most important questions posed to these fifty-six women who required hysterectomies was how they had prepared themselves for surgery, both mentally and physically. Had they arranged for help at home with meals, housework, and child care following surgery? Of those women who responded to the survey, only fourteen admitted to not having made any arrangements at all.

Nine of the fifty-six indicated they had either chosen to go it alone or that help had not been readily available. Linda reported, "I left the hospital after twenty-four hours, took a long walk five days later, and went jogging at three and a half weeks." Because of her unusual energy, spark, and refreshing outlook on life, Linda served as a model for others. She was also a breast cancer survivor.

Another commented that she, like me, had prepared meals in advance so that she felt she'd be able to "wing it alone."

Some managed to survive with just minimum help. In another case, the church brought in meals.

Others relied on family members and friends for help and support. Leading the list of supporters were husbands and boyfriends. Next in line for "active duty" came mothers and hired help. Third were sons and daughters, followed by close friends, then fathers. Three sets of in-laws pitched in, in lieu of absentee husbands, and, finally, a sister assisted one woman.

The actual survey materials are presented in the appendixes. The following statistics summarize initial findings from the survey:

1. *Age*

26–30	2
31–40	8
41–50	17
51–60	22
61–70	13
71–82	5
Unanswered	8

2. *Marital status*

Married	56
Single	4
Separated/divorced	8
Widowed	2
Unanswered	5

3. *Type of surgery*

Vaginal hysterectomy	5
Subtotal hysterectomy	6
Total hysterectomy	14
Total with bilateral salpingo-ovariectomy	17

Total with unilateral salpingo-ovariectomy	3
Radical hysterectomy	2
Myomectomy	7
Unanswered	11

4. *Conditions requiring surgery*

Bleeding	15
Tumors/fibroids	19
Prolapsed uterus	3
Malignancy	6
Precancer	8
Endometriosis	7
Cysts	5
Other (e.g., after multiple C-sections)	16

Those women for whom surgery was considered elective were then asked to comment on whether they felt the decision was justified by the outcome. Although a few declined to answer, only two women responded negatively. The first, a single woman just twenty-seven years old, was mourning her infertility. The second woman, who gave her age as "over sixty-five," stated that she never should have done it, although she did not elaborate. A third, whose hysterectomy took place ten years earlier, was uncertain about the necessity of her surgery because, as she said, "today there are more medical advances."

An overwhelming majority of all women surveyed (approximately 75 percent) also indicated that they had been fully informed about their condition. In addition, nearly 50 percent sought second and, in some cases, third and fourth opinions before proceeding with surgery. Only eleven people admitted that they had not been apprised of all the facts.

Almost half of the women surveyed encountered little to no difficulty regarding the physical changes following surgery. Eight reported noticing some change but dismissed it as relatively unimportant, and five commented on positive changes that included weight loss, the elimination of abdominal bloating, decreased frequency in urination, the end of menstruation, and the elimination of mood swings.

On the negative side, 25 percent of the women surveyed mentioned being distressed over unpleasant changes. Two women felt their bodies were changing and that they looked more "middle-aged," citing dry skin and hair, weight gain, hot flashes, and unsightly scars. Another woman experienced increased constipation, urination, and bloating. Still others commented mostly on fatigue and insomnia, loss of abdominal muscle tone, weight gain, and "disfiguring" scars.

It may be interesting to note that 50 percent of the women reported no change whatsoever in either their appetite or weight. Of the other 50 percent, twenty-three reported to have gained weight after surgery, thirteen reported weight loss, and three were uncertain. In some cases of weight gain, increased appetites were also noted. In other cases, it was the sudden change in body chemistry that was thought to have been responsible. Others blamed the problem on HRT.

The subject of HRT and ERT was a major consideration for everyone. Nevertheless, twice as many people as not in this study opted for some form of hormone therapy after surgery regardless of any possible risk factor. In most cases in which undesirable changes were observed, they appeared to be correlated with failure to use HRT.

Only a handful of all the women questioned (15 percent) reported to having any type of complication resulting from surgery. Three of the five mentioned postsurgical infections; one woman specifically blamed the hospital for having prematurely discharged her after only seventy-two hours. The most serious complication involved a nicked bladder, a problem that seldom occurs during a hysterectomy. This complication necessitated a second surgical procedure in which a catheter was inserted, and the patient had to wear a plastic bag for two months afterward.

Scarring was more of an issue for cancer patients because the incisions tend to be longer more noticeable vertical cuts that extend from the navel to the pubic bone. Conversely, the horizontal or Pfannestiel incision, known also as a bikini cut, is more discreet and results in less scarring. The bikini cut is only four to six inches long, located just above the pubic hairline, extending from hipbone to hipbone. It is interesting, however, that in our group of women the type of incision was very evenly divided between those who had bikini cuts and those with vertical incisions.

Regardless of any physical alterations to the body, a vast majority (two-thirds of those surveyed) said they did not suffer any trace of postsurgical depression. Of the remaining 33 percent who did suffer from depression, the reasons most frequently cited were a feeling of loss of womanhood and the inability to conceive, unexplained pain, a general feeling of lethargy, and a lack of support and understanding from husbands and other family members. Nevertheless, most of the women did recover with time, either on their own or with the help of professional guidance.

What seemed most encouraging was how the majority of people reflected on their quality of life since recovery. Comments were largely favorable although some women felt the quality of their lives had remained unchanged. One woman even said she felt younger, sexier, and "clean." Another commented, "Free at last!" Some felt that a hysterectomy was no big deal because they had survived greater tragedies.

"I had a friend going through the same thing, and for her it was a piece of cake."

Another said, "I had a mastectomy two months before, and my divorce was finalized the day before the mastectomy—this surgery was nothing!"

Thirty-three women responded very positively, emphasizing a good mental attitude prior to surgery. Some had even felt physically strong. Of those thirty-three, nine emphasized the importance of physical fitness.

"At first I was frightened at the thought of a major operation, but then realized that being physically fit would help me through the long recuperation period," said one woman who spoke with great candor and determination.

"I worked on a plan for almost a year," described another long-range planner. "I worked with a trainer, controlled my diet, and took lots of vitamins."

One person, a psychotherapist, had delayed her surgery for two months while she mentally prepared by using her knowledge of self-hypnosis (hypnotherapy) to help guide her through this period.

Another took a vacation, then spent time in the library reading everything she could find on the subject of uterine cancer. She also kept to her daily walk routine. Other women stressed *their* individual needs and their readiness.

What seemed most encouraging was how the majority of people reflected on their quality of life since recovery. Comments were largely favorable although some women felt the quality of their lives had remained unchanged.

"By the time I had surgery, I had been experiencing such bad periods that I was ready to have it already," exclaimed one woman with a sigh of relief.

"I had less than one month to prepare," responded someone who just recently had undergone a radical hysterectomy for cervical cancer. "I tried to postpone surgery because of my job and because I was also right in the middle of a project. I didn't think about myself—my work and my husband came first." Others sounded very matter-of-fact in their comments:

"My situation was life-threatening so I told myself I had to get through it."

"It had to be done!"

"Since there was a problem that needed corrective measures, I looked forward to the surgery."

"I just wanted to get it over with."

Only a few of the women who were interviewed in depth seemed unhappy with their lives postsurgically, and usually this view was related to a less satisfying sex life.

Four expressed serious doubts they had confronted prior to surgery. These are the women you've met in Chapters 9 and 10.

"My husband and I talked about it," said Karen. "He had some really male concerns. The idea that I would no longer be able to have children was a problem for him even though we already had three healthy kids. Then, my own concern: Who am I going to be?"

"I was very worried and frightened," remarked someone else. "I tried to think positively."

Five people admittedly had no time to think about anything beforehand because they had been rushed into surgery:

"It was Christmas time," said Ann. "I didn't have time to think and worry about it. I decided on the Monday after Thanksgiving, and surgery was scheduled for December 27. I had one bad day after I had made the decision to go ahead with it. I felt very depressed and feared a lack of femininity and the loss of sexuality."

"I saw my doctor on a Wednesday," began Stephanie. "He insisted upon my having surgery on that very Friday—my fiftieth birthday! He said I couldn't wait another week, which was very upsetting. I felt railroaded."

On the other hand, others looked on their surgery as a turning point—a time of personal growth, a chance to redefine priorities and to take better care of their health.

"I read a lot of books and prayed a lot," commented Pat, the twenty-seven-year-old still in mourning over her infertility.

"I said lots of prayers and listened to the voice from within."

"After seeing my doctor, I spoke with our minister," said another.

Nine of the women interviewed in depth had prepared themselves by doing some thorough research:

"Physically I felt somewhat weak since I had had three D&C's plus two hysteroscopies, all within the space of five months," said Carol. "I prepared myself mentally by attending yoga classes, doing lots of reading and research, and I listened to audiocassettes on relaxation and preparing for surgery. I also worked with a therapist and someone from HERS [Hysterectomy Educational Resources and Services]."

HERS is a national not-for-profit resource organization for educational information on hysterectomy. After Carol phoned the organization, she was instructed to write a letter detailing her condition. Carol's letter was then forwarded to ten women with similar experiences who lived nearby. Not only did these other women provide an empathetic ear, but Carol then had someone to talk with who understood and shared her plight. From this list of ten women Carol made a life-long friend who lives in New York.

For information regarding women's resource groups in your area, consult the community service pages of your local telephone book. You can also contact HERS:

HERS Foundation
Hysterectomy Educational Resources and Services
422 Bryn Mawr Avenue
Bala Cynwyd, PA 19004
Phone: (610) 667-7757
Fax: (610) 667-8096
Web site: *www.dca.net/~hers/net*
E-mail: *HERSFdn@aol.com*

PEOPLE WHO have difficulty adapting to change will likely have trouble with any changes that follow hysterectomy. But regardless of your capability to adjust, it is important to maintain an open and positive attitude. Although you may hear of horror stories—women who were physically mangled and sexually destroyed—these cases are extremely uncommon. As you read on, you will learn that the vast majority of women in this survey reported no effect on their sexual functioning, and nearly one-half reported some improvement. Only nine of the seventy-five women reported any negative consequences, either sexually or otherwise.

CHAPTER THIRTEEN

WOMEN'S WORKSHOP: "THE SUCCESSFUL MILLENNIUM WOMAN—a STRONG MIND, BODY, and SOUL"

MY POSTHYSTERECTOMY experience led me to create a women's workshop, divided into five separate sessions and available to all participants of the survey. I wanted not only to help women cope after surgery, but also to attempt to reach out to those with presurgical conditions. The purpose was for women to feel safe in a nonthreatening environment so they could freely discuss their individual problems with others. The workshop would be run in similar fashion to a support group, and the results would be carefully analyzed and later documented. The identities of all participants would remain strictly confidential, and people would also be requested not to discuss anything outside the room that took place during the meetings.

OPENING SESSION

The day finally arrived for the gathering of our first workshop. Many of us were strangers to one another, knowing each other only well enough to casually greet hello. What I soon discovered, however, was how freely women express themselves when alone together without the presence of men. An interesting exchange of ideas flourished, which were sparked still further by one dissenting voice playing devil's advocate, Judy.

Soon a lively discussion began on the subject "HRT, yes or no?" What are the short- and long-term effects of estrogen replacement? Women complained about weight gain and their fears of someday developing cancer after years of having taken hormones. Janis wondered whether HRT might have been responsible for her having contracted uterine cancer at fifty-five.

"I had not had my period for six months when my doctor prescribed estrogen patch and progesterone," said Janis.

Linda was advised not to take ERT since she was a breast cancer survivor, but Karen used both progesterone and estrogen creams even though her mother and maternal grandmother had died from ovarian cancer.

We discussed the various benefits of ERT:[1]

- offers relief from hot flashes,
- retards aging of the skin by helping preserve moisture and toning,
- prevents premature vaginal atrophy while restoring moisture and flexibility,
- helps prevent bladder infections caused by estrogen deficiency,
- helps avoid osteoporosis,
- protects against heart disease by lowering cholesterol and improving the cardiovascular system,
- reduces headaches by dilating blood vessels, and
- (still unproven) may also help women in later life avoid rheumatoid arthritis.

ERT may also reduce the risk of developing Alzheimer's disease as well as making the symptoms of the disease milder in those cases where it has already developed.[2]

Some of the women seemed hopeful that ERT might prevent them from the ravages of aging such as dry, wrinkled skin. Someone else even mentioned the theory that ERT increases breast size. That comment brought down the house! The cancer victims, however, were happy just to be alive. The big question: how long can women stay on ERT? Ten years, fifteen years, forever? What are the alternatives to conventional HRT, and are they effective?

In the middle of this interesting exchange I could see Judy smoldering in the first row. When her turn came to speak she exploded, vehemently protesting the dangers of HRT and ERT.

"Don't you realize that hormones are responsible for the epidemic of breast and uterine cancer? No personal baseline levels have been established at thirty-five, forty, forty-five, et cetera. It's appalling that tens of thousands of women are on the exact same dosage, particularly since cancer is a side effect. No bone scans are performed. No monitoring of the replacement hormone levels has been established. Hormones are prescribed like aspirin. Doctors are promoting the pharmaceutical companies, and they're probably getting big kickbacks!

"My grandmother had a mastectomy in her fifties. My mother had a radical mastectomy at forty-eight, but by that time her cancer had already metastasized and she died two years later. Then my aunt went on ERT ten years ago, my mother's youngest sister. I pleaded with her not to take it; two months ago she had a hysterectomy. Uterine cancer. How many more people have to die before ERT and HRT are taken off the market?"

Suddenly everyone burst into an uproar. No one seemed to agree with Judy, and for a few moments I felt uncomfortable. Although Judy's concerns were valid, this topic unquestionably was a volatile issue. It was particularly inflammatory because cancer survivors were present, not to mention Gladys, who had been operated on just six days earlier. Fortunately, Mary, as a nurse in a doctor's office, was able to speak for the other side. Though I still worried whether Mary's comments were sufficient to quell the unrest after Judy's vehement arguments, it was nevertheless a healthy exchange.

HRT has been known to elicit the following short-term side effects: fluid retention, nausea, irritability, and tension. Excessively high dosages of estrogen can lead to breast tenderness. However, these side effects usually disappear after a couple months. Bear in mind that any kind of hormonal replacement has benefits as well as side effects—it is not a panacea.

Other supplemental hormonal combinations are often prescribed as well, such as estrogen and androgen (a hormone present in both sexes but more so in males). However, estrogen and androgen have been reported to produce such masculine characteristics as facial and body hair growth and deepening of the voice.

To prevent giving HRT to any woman who might be at risk to a particular disease, the Food and Drug Administration (FDA) has developed a list of contraindications to HRT: thrombosis, breast cancer, liver involvement, and gallbladder disease.[3]

To prevent giving HRT to any woman who might be at risk to a particular disease, the Food and Drug Administration (FDA) has developed a list of contraindications to HRT: thrombosis, breast cancer, liver involvement, and gallbladder disease.

SESSION 2: DR. MARTIN KASS

"Dr. Kass, I promised you last September that one day you'd be so famous that women would be lined up waiting at your office door just for the opportunity to schedule their hysterectomies." Everyone laughed, including Dr. Kass, who was seated to my right and smiling good-naturedly. "Some of them have even come to meet you this evening," I chuckled, "and I also see a few of your own patients who can attest to your superb surgical expertise."

Both the audience and Dr. Kass seemed to be enjoying this moment with me. But where was Ann, I wondered? I couldn't imagine her not attending tonight's meeting, especially with her own doctor scheduled to speak. Quickly I glanced in his direction, then continued.

"One of your patients unfortunately seems to be missing tonight, but last week she described her surgical scar to me as looking like a 'smiling face.'" He nodded, obviously aware of whom I was speaking.

Scanning the room very quickly, I noticed Judy's absence, too. I had spoken with her after last week's meeting and knew that she had felt "attacked," as if everyone had been against her. I had tried to explain that it wasn't what she had said but, perhaps, how she had expressed her opinions that had triggered the reaction from other women.

Judy was nonetheless unhappy. She believed that if she were the only one so fiercely opposed to HRT, then she had no business being there. Nobody understood her. She felt alone; no one cared, or seemed to have the slightest interest in what she thought. "They won't accept the truth," she had stated, with blatant discomfort.

Once more, I had tried to persuade Judy to return. "Why not raise your concerns next week with Dr. Kass?" I suggested. "After all, you asked the questions that others were too afraid to ask."

"What's the point?" she had defiantly responded. "He'll be pushing estrogen just like everyone else."

"I'M HERE to learn from you," began Dr. Kass. He directed our attention to the clipboard on which he began to diagram a sketch of a woman's lower anatomy. "Several procedures are used today in performing hysterectomies," he continued. "The decision of which one to use is determined first by the nature of the problem, and then it is up to the doctor's discretion as to which technique best suits the needs of his or her patient.

"Many women prefer a vaginal hysterectomy performed because there's no visible incision. Sometimes it's possible, but not in cases that involve large fibroids, and, definitely not when we're suspicious of a carcinoma. The problem with the vaginal procedure is in not being able to see well enough to thoroughly examine the abdominal cavity. Also, there's no room to vaginally remove large fibroids.

"A fairly new technique is laparoscopically assisted vaginal surgery. With this procedure a small incision is first made at the patient's belly button, then several other small cuts are made before clamping off the uterus and removing it vaginally. Personally, I don't like the procedure because there's no depth perception.

"An abdominal hysterectomy can be done by either making a horizontal incision, better known as a bikini cut, or a vertical one. The bikini incision, which I know most of you prefer because it's less noticeable, is actually a much stronger one. It's very rare to have an incisional hernia after this type of incision, and it's also easier to separate the abdominal muscles without severing them. This is the method I usually recommend to patients with large fibroids, uterine prolapse, and also endometriosis."

Uterine prolapse is the abnormal protrusion of the uterus through the pelvic floor. The muscular structure of the uterus can weaken, particularly after multiple births. If a woman's level of estrogen is insufficient, this condition can cause the uterus to drop down and sag into the wall of the vagina. In extreme cases, the uterus can be seen to protrude from between the legs.

A prolapsed uterus must be corrected because it will continue to worsen until repaired. Besides being uncomfortable, it can cause urinary incontinence by weakening the bladder.[4]

Just then a hand went up in the front row. It was Stephanie. "Dr. Kass, you know about my case," she said. "I had large fibroids, too. Why couldn't I have had a bikini incision instead of the very large and ugly vertical one I was given? I was shocked when I woke up after surgery and saw where I had been cut. I couldn't imagine what had happened." Nodding compassionately, Dr. Kass responded.

"We refer to large fibroids as being grapefruit size. But there are different size grapefruits. Some are easily removable with a horizontal incision, but others are too big. In that case, there isn't enough space to take them out through a bikini opening. Yours, I believe, was one of the larger fibroids that needed to be removed vertically." Although Stephanie understood him, she didn't seem quite convinced.

"Although we normally prefer to remove the cervix as a preventive measure against cervical cancer, which is deadly," continued Dr. Kass, "some women do feel that it adds to their sexual enjoyment and they want to keep their cervix. With a vaginal hysterectomy there's no option; the cervix is automatically removed.

"With younger women still in their childbearing years, we prefer to leave the uterus intact and only remove the fibroid itself. This is what is commonly referred to as a myomectomy. The down side of this procedure is that fibroids oftentimes grow back and then these women end up returning at a later date anyway for a hysterectomy. We try to avoid the need for the second operation, if possible.

"Now, when there's evidence of cancer, a radical hysterectomy is performed through a vertical incision. Not only does this involve a total hysterectomy, but also lymph nodes as well as other surrounding tissue is removed to help increase the odds of survival. Sometimes this is followed by radiation therapy when doctors feel the cancer may have spread."

According to *The Harvard Guide to Women's Health,* a woman with stage 1 cancer may be treated with radiation depending on her risk for recurrence of the disease. This determination is based upon the size of the tumor and whether it has permeated the uterine wall. If the disease is minimal, radiation is not necessary.

Stage 2 carcinoma is almost always treated with radiation since the cancer has spread to nearby lymph nodes. Stage 3 carcinoma is treated even more aggressively, sometimes requiring extensive abdominal radiation. If the cancer has advanced to stage 4, or if an earlier carcinoma has recurred after the conclusion of radiation treatment, hormone therapy or chemotherapy is oftentimes advised.[5]

Dr. Kass described the high-risk category for developing cancer: you have a family history of cancer, you have had a previous other cancer, you have had abnormal Pap smears, you have genital herpes or warts, you take birth control pills, and/or you smoke.

It is believed that lifestyle does play an important factor in determining a woman's chances of cervical cancer. If a young woman had sexual intercourse before or during puberty, she may be in a more vulnerable position. A higher degree of vulnerability exists at puberty because the cervix is undergoing significant changes then. A woman also increases her risk of cancer if she has multiple sexual partners and does not insist on the use of condoms.[6]

Appearing again as a big issue in this session, as in the first, was estrogen as well as other hormone replacement therapy.

"Today it is commonly advised to offer ERT even to those women who have recovered from operations involving the removal of malignant tumors, with the exception of breast cancer," said Dr. Kass. "Estrogen can now be prescribed as a viable option between two months and two years following surgery because many doctors strongly feel the risks are far greater for developing other serious problems without the use of ERT. Statistically, for example, we know that more women die of heart disease each year than from cancer," he emphasized. This theory has also been supported by data collected by the U.S. government in 1980. Research carried out that year to determine the causes of death of postmenopausal women came up with the following results: 485,000 women died from cardiovascular disease, 38,400 from breast cancer, 20,525 from diabetes mellitus, 12,225 from hypertension, 11,600 from ovarian cancer, 6,800 from cervical cancer, and 2,900 from uterine cancer.[7]

"What is also significant," continued Dr. Kass, "is that although 30 percent of all women will develop fibroids during their lifetime, only one out of a thousand of these fibroids will actually become malignant. Ovarian cancer, on the other hand, is more deadly. One out of seventy ovarian tumors is malignant. But I know the biggest scare for most of you is breast cancer." Nobody there disagreed. Yet even on this issue Dr. Kass offered some encouraging news as he went on to illustrate the study that has been tracking fifty thousand female nurses over the past fifteen years.

"Already there have been some early, yet inconclusive, results," said Dr. Kass, "as it appears that only after age sixty are women at a 10 to 15 percent greater risk of developing breast cancer than those women who have not used ERT. But the final verdict is still not in since the nurses will continue to be tracked for the rest of their lives.

"My own close examination of twenty-three studies revealed no increased risk of breast cancer. When a slight elevation of risk was noticed, it was usually not until after ERT had been taken for fifteen or more years. Women on HRT are usually more closely monitored than nonusers because they receive regular checkups. Biannual breast examinations and mammograms offer early detection in screening for breast cancer."

"What is also significant," continued Dr. Kass, "is that although 30 percent of all women will develop fibroids during their lifetime, only one out of a thousand of these fibroids will actually become malignant."

In the nurses' study, to which Dr. Kass referred, there was a 28 to 32 percent increase in risk for breast cancer in women who took estrogen for five years or more and were still using ERT. Even more notable, one month after the data from the nurse's study had been released, the University of Washington came out with its own findings. Researchers there found no increase in breast cancer in women who took estrogen for twenty years. In March 1996 the American Cancer Society (ACS) published its research after having followed more than 420,000 women from 1982 to 1992. The ACS also found no increase in cancer risk for women who had been taking estrogen pills for more than ten years. In fact, an overall 16 percent decrease in breast cancer mortality existed for women who had taken estrogen at any time in their life.[8]

Regardless of hormone therapy being a highly controversial issue about which everyone seemed to have her own opinions,

Dr. Kass was questioned about his recommendations. "As with the use of any hormones, HRT is a personal decision," he responded. "Women concerned about the aging process almost invariably want ERT since estrogen is what keeps women looking and feeling young and healthy. It is widely known that loss of estrogen not only can lead to dry, wrinkled skin but also to vaginal dryness. Vaginal dryness is a common symptom in postmenopausal women since levels of estrogen diminish as the body ages."

Several women admitted to having similar experiences because of not using an estrogen supplement. Janis remained a dissenting voice.

"I wanted only to celebrate life!" she exclaimed. "It didn't matter the kind of incision I had or what was removed—I wanted to live." So did the other cancer survivors who were present; they all just wanted to live.

Natalie spoke up next. "I felt as if I had been lied to about my libido. For six to eight weeks after surgery I felt nothing." Dr. Kass didn't seem surprised by Natalie's experience.

"This is something you should discuss next week with Dr. Metres, the psychologist."

Dr. Kass's closing remarks dealt with other brands of estrogen on the market. He tends more frequently to prescribe Premarin because it's the only natural form of estrogen. "Premarin," he said, "is made from the urine of pregnant horses. All other estrogen replacements are synthetics."

"But what about the patch?" asked Janis.

"We have greater flexibility in adjusting the dosage of estrogen pills. With the patch you can't really adjust it," he replied.

A final question, concerning Premarin vaginal cream, was addressed by Dr. Kass. "That may be a good product," he said, "but it must be kept in mind that any estrogen vaginal cream is inadequate in helping to prevent osteoporosis or heart disease."

Hormonal vaginal cream does little to prevent osteoporosis or heart disease because of its low level of absorption into the blood stream—approximately one-half to one-quarter of the strength that a woman receives from taking estrogen in pill form.[9]

Women who suffer from vaginal dryness, however, will benefit from Premarin cream. Applied topically every day to the genital area, the cream will decrease dryness, if not reverse vaginal atrophy. Kegel exercises (used to strengthen genital muscles; described later in this chapter) and frequent intercourse (or masturbation) will also help diminish vaginal dryness.[10]

Keep in mind, too, that vaginal cream is not effective for hot flashes (or flushes). Hot flashes can best be minimized by avoiding potential problems, such as stress, hot weather, warm rooms, hot drinks, alcohol, caffeine, and spicy foods.[11]

SESSION 3: DR. PHIL METRES

Speaking at the next workshop session was Dr. Phil Metres, a licensed clinical psychologist specializing in individual counseling, marital counseling, and family therapy.

Dr. Metres began, "I enjoyed Dr. Kass's opening remark last week when he said, 'I'm here to learn from you.' I'm also here to learn from you since I'm operating out of ignorance and want to learn. I have read about hysterectomies, and I want to listen carefully.

"Men are very different from women in the way they think and react to situations, like John Gray described in his book *Men Are from Mars, Women Are from Venus.* As men we need to fix things, but we don't always know how to express our feelings. We need to listen, not just fix.

"The study of gynecological medicine is generally pursued by those interested not only in research, but in clinical treatment as well. Medical students in this field tend to be compulsive, highly competitive individuals who later become busy doctors, some of whom may also have a tendency to remain detached from their patients. Unfortunately, instances of greed and robotization induced by training and sleepless residency nights may have an impact on otherwise normal doctor-patient relationships. Since doctors often have knowledge and experience in life and death matters, it's very human to regard them as the father figure, God, the Law."

Out of the corner of my eye I spotted Judy. I was glad she had returned for another session—and even seemed to be enjoying it. It seemed that I had misinterpreted the feelings of the other women who had been present at our first session. Several had approached me after our second meeting with Dr. Kass, wondering why Judy had not returned. "She added spark," I was told, "and she was fun." I phoned to inform her that she had been missed.

"The women want to hear controversial opinions," I had said. "You need to show up next week; please don't disappoint us. Everyone's counting on you."

"WHAT I realize," continued Dr. Metres, "is that many women reach their peak years during their fifties, whereas men begin declining at this time as their level of testosterone decreases. Women, it seems, actually release a burst of energy and creative power. It is a time to develop their own individuality and talents. Yet, when a woman is faced with hysterectomy during this stage of life, she's more vulnerable to emotional and psychological problems because her very womanhood is threatened. The loss of the uterus can lead to a sharp decrease in sexual pleasure, sometimes bringing on what we call a clinical depression.

"Clinical depression is recognizable by one or more of the following symptoms: (1) marked change in weight (five pounds—up or down), (2) excessive guilt, (3) sleep disorders, (4) feelings of lifelessness, (5) loss of libido, (6) lack of concentration, (7) memory loss, and (8) a pervasive sense of worthlessness or guilt." He stopped and looked from face to face, waiting for feedback.

Ann spoke up. "Before my operation my husband thought my complaints were mostly psychological. He didn't understand. He had no idea that a hysterectomy meant major surgery. Not until Dr. Kass sat down to explain things to him did he first begin to realize what I was going through.

"I told one doctor off in the hospital last week, and he sent in a psychiatrist." Now all eyes were riveted upon Ann. "Yes," said she, "and he called me a hypo-maniac." Everyone sat a little straighter to listen. It was now obviously why she hadn't been present last week—Ann had been hospitalized.

"In the middle of the night I awakened in a lot of pain and went to the hospital emergency room. My husband and I sat there for what seemed like hours while they waited for the doctor on call to phone in. Finally I was admitted. The next morning, when my internist arrived to see me, I was so angry that I told him off." Ann looked serious. "That's when he called in the psychiatrist."

"But, Ann," interjected Mary, "by law a doctor has only thirty minutes to get to the hospital if he's on call. Otherwise there can be a lawsuit."

"I suppose we could have sued," replied Ann, pensively. "But so much was happening, and now it's after the fact. For six days and nights I lay in my hospital bed while I was worked over from head to toe by more doctors and nurses than I could count. It had nothing to do with the hysterectomy, and Dr. Kass was called in only as a consultant. I have arthritic legs and a hip, and there was inflammation of the groin." She winced as she spoke.

"A hysterectomy can be overpowering if you aren't used to paying attention to your body," commented Mary. "It's body and mind—the total entity."

"That's right," said Dr. Metres, "and at this critical time some people also find themselves at odds with their HMOs. It becomes a real problem, sometimes causing untold anguish and grief when a woman needs permission from her primary care agency before she can even proceed with required surgery."

It was Janis's turn next. "I had cancer. My problem was not about facing major surgery, even knowing there was a malignancy, but it was the dread of being put to sleep under a general anesthesia. I was petrified."

"Let's talk for a moment about the 'Big C,'" said Dr. Metres, eyeing Janis compassionately as he sensed her conflict. "How do you feel when threatened with cancer? What are your first reactions to such frightening news?"

"What bothered me most was that my own doctor would not listen to me," said Janis. "He was adamant about putting me through a general anesthesia despite my fear. Had it not been for a very considerate and understanding anesthesiologist whom I convinced to give me an epidural, I would have been confronted not only with cancer, but also the fear of dying on the operating table."

"Those are powerful and very real concerns," replied Dr. Metres. "The very nature of healing comes from the caring relationship between a doctor and his patient. Perhaps it's time to consider the meaning of spirituality. Spiritual thoughts and feelings may emerge as part of the healing process from hysterectomy. If we put aside the actual surgery for a moment, how do you feel about knowing that you can't bear children any more?"

Beth responded first. "I was already in my fifties when I had surgery, but even though I didn't want more children, knowing I couldn't have children was depressing."

"Some men are jealous of a woman's natural ability to nurture life within her own body and then bond more easily with that child," responded Dr. Metres. "It is parallel to penis envy in women." A muffled twitter was overheard.

"Frankly," exclaimed Judy, "I wouldn't mind unzipping this thing," as she pointed to her abdomen, "and getting rid of it."

An uproar, of sorts, ensued. Some of us may still have been reflecting over Dr. Metres's previous observation when Judy finished her statement.

"But that's me!" said she. "How many of you know that over a certain age—forty-seven, I think—it is protocol for doctors to take out everything—uterus, ovaries, even the appendix must go."

"No!" shouted Mary. "Those decisions are made on an individual basis, and not until the patient reaches the OR. That's untrue!"

"Insurance companies don't want to pay twice," insisted Judy.

"Not true," Mary repeated.

"It is necessary to sign a release," interjected Dr. Metres.

"Yes. There's an operative report that says everything—possible oophorectomy, possible appendectomy," answered Mary.

"Even so," added Dr. Metres, "if something were taken away against my will, it would have spiritual implications. It takes time to deal with this. Let's pause for a moment to reconsider the doctor-patient relationship. Take your case, Stephanie. I think it would be appropriate for you to speak with your doctor about why and how he did what he did to you, and your feelings about this." Stephanie nodded, without a moment's pause.

> *"Not everyone has had kids, or wants kids, but a hysterectomy is final. There's that wish to generate life and, perhaps, to continue to generate life even beyond child bearing years. Then there's subsequent grief, regardless of age."*

"We need to sum up," announced Dr. Metres at last. "I'd like to close this evening's session focusing in upon the spiritual implications of hysterectomy. Not everyone has had kids, or wants kids, but a hysterectomy is final. There's that wish to generate life and, perhaps, to continue to generate life even beyond child bearing years. Then there's subsequent grief, regardless of age.

"Reduce your sense of time and urgency. Move more slowly. Find time and space for yourself. Eat; pray, reach out to God or to your higher power, and feel that power reaching back to you.

"Many roads lead to God," said Dr. Metres, speaking reflectively. As he paused, one could sense his deep emotion.

"We all have different ways of reaching ourselves. We can learn new things when we put our minds and hearts to it. There remains a mystery in all of life, and in all of us individually and collectively."

SESSION 4: KAREN BROWNLEE AND FERN RITACCA

Personal trainer Karen Brownlee entered and began our session on physical fitness. "When Dr. Kass addressed us two weeks ago, we learned that abdominal muscles are rarely severed during a hysterectomy, only separated. If these muscles are not cut, then it's possible to regain full muscular control. Not only do most women want to tighten up those abdominal muscles and flatten their stomachs, but there are other even more important reasons for working abdominal muscles. Good muscular control can alleviate and even prevent urinary incontinence, a problem for many older women; diminished sexual function; and genital prolapse."

Karen described the type of exercise beneficial to women recovering not only from hysterectomy surgery, but also from postpartum cesarean delivery.

"There are exercises designed for each stage of recovery," she told the group.

"The first set of exercises, immediate recovery exercises, can begin only after you first discuss this with your doctor. Then, with your physician's permission to start moving again, you can begin to incorporate the following exercises."

Immediate recovery exercises maintain lung capacity and prevent pulmonary complications. They also help to maintain muscle tonicity and promote circulation, especially to the lower extremities. These initial recovery exercises also help to facilitate recovery time. Karen then demonstrated the following exercises:

Deep breathing: Inhale deeply through your nose; exhale by blowing slowly through mouth with lips slightly separated.

Isometric abdominals: Lying on your back with your knees bent, inhale deeply letting your abdomen expand, and hold for five seconds. Exhale completely while pulling in the abdomen.

Ankles: Point and flex feet, and make circles in both directions.

Isometric thigh and buttocks: Cross your ankles; tighten all muscles in your legs, knees, thighs, and buttocks; and hold for five seconds; relax.

Arms and shoulders: Shrug and circle backward each shoulder separately. Raise and lower each arm. Gently reach overhead (it may be helpful to support the incision with your free hand).

Next are early recovery exercises, which help restore normal body movement, especially the midsection. Depending on how you feel and what your doctor says, these exercises may be started within twenty-four hours following surgery. Repeat each exercise as tolerated, with adequate rest in between.

Lying alternate knee bends: Lying on your back with one leg outstretched and the other knee bent up with your foot on bed, slide the heel of the bent leg down to the straight leg's foot and back up to the bent-knee position. Repeat for both legs.

Rolling side to side: While relaxing abdominals, use your arms and shoulders to roll yourself from one side to the other; gently roll your legs along with your upper body.

Getting in/out of bed: Lying on your side, bend your knees up and slide your feet to the edge of the bed. Push up with your arms to a sitting position, using one hand to support your incision if necessary. Breathe deeply and slide your legs over the edge of the bed, gently swinging your feet several times. Using the bedside for support, take another deep breath, then tighten your buttocks and abdominals while gradually putting your weight down on your feet. (If necessary, use a footstool so you don't have to reach that far.)

Sitting down in a chair: Select an arm chair; you may also want to have pillows arranged along the back of the chair so you are sitting close to the edge. With your back to the chair, scoot the back of your legs against the seat of the chair. Reach behind you and put your hand on the arm of the chair (you may want the other hand on your incision for support). Gently lean forward and lower yourself into the seat with your weight on your arm(s) and your legs.

Getting out of a chair: Put one or both hands on the arm(s) of the chair (you may want one hand on your incision to support it), and slide all the way up to the edge of the seat.

Gently lean forward and push up with your hand(s) and legs.

Walking: Look forward rather than down at the floor. Stand as straight as you can, gently pulling in the lower abdominal muscles to give better support to the incision area.

Second-day exercises continue to enhance blood flow throughout the body while improving your midsection mobility. Repeat these several times throughout the day:

Isometric buttocks/inner thigh: Lying on your back, bend your knees up and place a pillow between them. Inhale, contract your buttocks, and squeeze the pillow for a count of ten. Exhale and relax. Work up to ten repetitions.

Pelvic tilt: Lying on your back with your knees up and feet flat, exhale and press your lower back into the floor/bed by contracting your abdominal and buttock muscles. Gently rock from a pelvic tilt (exhale) to a relaxed position (inhale).

Upper abdominal kneading: Just below your breasts, knead your abdomen to help move gas along your digestive tract and aid in elimination.

Knees to side: Lying on your back with your knees up and feet flat, exhale and slowly lower both knees to one side. Inhale while bringing your knees back up to the start position, and then repeat on the other side.

Tigney knee extension: Lying on your back, extend your legs straight out and push the back of your knees into the bed, tightening your thigh muscles. Hold for a count of five.

Isometric glute squeeze: Lying on your back with extended legs, tighten your buttocks and hold for a count of five.

Several days of postsurgery exercises will further strengthen your abdominal muscles. Once you can comfortably tolerate the preceding exercises, your doctor will graduate you so you may then proceed on with this next set of exercises:

Pectoral push: Raise the head of the bed, or with several pillows behind your shoulders and head, sit up carefully. Put your palms together in front of your chest, exhale, and press your palms into each other. Inhale and relax; repeat.

Pelvic bridge: Lying on your back with your knees bent, feet flat, arms at your sides and a pillow under your head, exhale while you tighten your abdomen and buttocks. Gently and slowly raise your hips off the bed. When you can raise your hips so you have a straight line from your knees to your shoulders, hold that position and gently twist your hips to the right and then to the left. Lower your buttocks to the bed and relax.

Modified abdominal curl: Lying in an inclined position either with the bed raised or several pillows under your shoulders and head, bend your knees up with your feet flat, tuck your chin in, and relax and breathe deeply. Reach your arms out in front of you and exhale while contracting your abdominal muscles and reaching for your knees. Be sure to lift only your head and shoulders (do not curl all the way up).

The next stage of exercises, one to two weeks postsurgery exercises (to be continued over the months to come), strengthen abdominal musculature, promote and restore proper postural alignment, and establish awareness of proper body mechanics. Start with five and increase to twenty-five repetitions per day.

Pelvic tilt: Lying on your back with your knees bent, feet flat, and arms at your sides, note the natural arch in your back. Using your abdominal and buttocks muscles, flatten out the arch in your back and push your back to the floor. Hold for a count of five while exhaling, and then inhale and relax.

Pelvic tilt with abdominal curl: Lying on your back with your knees bent, feet flat and in a pelvic tilt position, reach your arms out in front of you and curl up, raising your head and shoulders. Slowly uncurl and release the pelvic tilt.

Pelvic tilt with external oblique abdominal curl: Lying on your back with your knees bent, feet flat and in a pelvic tilt position, place your left hand on your bottom-most right rib. Reach out with your right hand toward your left knee while raising your head and shoulders from the floor as you curl up. With your left hand, try to feel the muscles on the right ribs (external obliques) as you sit up. Slowly uncurl and release the pelvic tilt. Repeat for the other side.

Straight leg raise: Lying on your back with one knee bent and feet flat, extend your arms straight down your sides. While doing an abdominal curl, extend your right hand down to your right ankle to contract the muscle on your right side between the outside of your rib cage and your hip bone (internal oblique). Repeat for the other side.

Lifting technique: Lift objects by bending your knees and hips and sticking your buttocks out behind you (avoid bending at the waist because it strains your lower back). Keep objects close to your body as you lift them, keep your chest up, and let your legs do most of the work.

FERN RITACCA, an expert on osteoporosis, spoke to us next.

"Osteoporosis is not a natural part of aging," began Fern. "It's called 'the disease of the nineties,' and scientists are now spending ten billion a year in trying to find a possible cure. Osteoporosis, or porous bones, is a systemic skeletal disease characterized by low bone mass. Gradually, as our bones begin to lose their natural supply of calcium and other minerals, they become less dense and more susceptible to fractures.

"As women we are four times more susceptible to this disease than men, especially postmenopausal women who have small skeletal frames. For this reason Caucasian and Asian women are the most susceptible groups, whereas it is conjectured that African Americans and Hispanics are least likely to be stricken since they usually have a denser bone structure."

The National Osteoporosis Foundation reported that 25 million Americans were afflicted with this crippling disease in 1991. It strikes more than half of all women over the age of sixty-five, with four of every five persons with osteoporosis being female. Usually there are no warning signals until a fracture occurs, most commonly in the hip, spine, or wrist. Sometimes fractured ribs can occur just from coughing. Osteoporosis is a preventable disease. It is best to build healthy bones during childhood and early adulthood, then continuing to strengthen them throughout life.

The National Osteoporosis Foundation reported that 25 million Americans were afflicted with this crippling disease in 1991. It strikes more than half of all women over the age of sixty-five, with four of every five persons with osteoporosis being female.

Although the causes of osteoporosis are still unknown, it is possible to determine who is at greater risk so preventative measures can be taken. A list of questions, developed by the National Osteoporosis Foundation, can help you determine your risk factor:

1. Do you have a small thin frame, or are you Caucasian or Asian?
2. Do you have a family history of osteoporosis?
3. Are you a postmenopausal woman?
4. Have you had an early or surgically induced menopause?
5. Have you been taking excessive thyroid medication or high doses of cortisone-like drugs for asthma, arthritis, or cancer?
6. Is your diet low in dairy products and other sources of calcium?
7. Are you physically inactive?
8. Do you smoke cigarettes or drink alcohol in excess?

The more yes answers you have, the greater your risk of developing the disease. It is important to check with your doctor and contact the national foundation for more information:

The National Osteoporosis Foundation
2100 M Street, NW, Suite 602
Washington, D.C. 20037

"Although children stop growing in height during their teenage years, bone density continues to form until most of us reach our late twenties," Fern told us. "Once peak bone mass has been attained, it stabilizes for several years until we're in our late thirties or forties. At the onset of menopause, the time when our menstrual periods stop, we can lose between 2 and 5 percent of bone mass each year for the first five years following menopause. Afterwards, about 1 percent of bone mass is lost each year unless a daily regime of estrogen, calcium, and exercise become part of a woman's daily life. Postmenopausal women, those who went through natural menopause as well as those who were surgically induced, are at high risk. These women can lose from 20 to 30 percent of their bone mass during the first five years after menopause. Since osteoporosis is also a genetic disease, postmenopausal women with a family history are at the greatest risk. However, there is hope, ladies, because in recent years medical interventions have been found to counteract this disease and in some cases even reverse the condition."

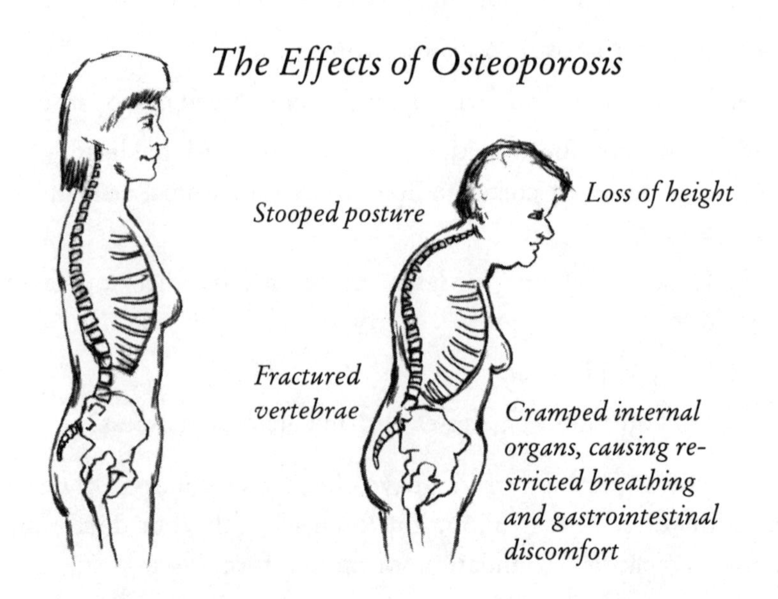

"For those of us not on estrogen," questioned Beth, "are there any nonhormonal drugs on the market?"

"Yes," replied Fern. "Merck has recently put out a new drug called Fosamax. Fosamax is a bisphosphonate, which is a drug used to reverse the progression of osteoporosis, and it actually helps to increase bone density in some people. In cases of low density, Fosamax can even be supplemented by women taking ERT. There are other drugs, such as Calcitonin, which are also available, but it's best to discuss this issue with your doctor. Some of these drugs may have a side effect, such as stomach upsets."

Another hand went up. This time, it was a woman who had been unable to attend the previous three sessions. Trudy, a woman in her late fifties, had two years earlier given her family one of the most beautiful gifts imaginable: a grandchild. For years her daughter had tried unsuccessfully to carry a pregnancy to term, so with the help of in vitro fertilization Trudy became impregnated with her own daughter's child and nine months later gave birth to a healthy baby girl. She had not had a hysterectomy and was experiencing problems with vaginal bleeding as a result of her late-in-life pregnancy.

"What kind of tests determine bone density?" asked Trudy.

"Bone density testing is administered by clinicians both at hospitals and special clinics," responded Fern. "The most accurate tests measure the total bone content of our hips, spine, and forearm. Other tests that measure the total calcium and mineral content of the hip and spine give off more radiation."

"What about Tums?" asked Beth. "I've heard that it's the same thing as taking calcium pills." Two other women in the group also reported taking Tums as a substitute for calcium.

"I've heard about that, too, Beth," replied Fern. "If you find you're receiving an adequate supply of calcium from what you're eating and using Tums only as a supplement, then continue.

"Both premenopausal and postmenopausal women who exercise can reduce the risk of osteoporosis. A good fitness program is a must for all of us," emphasized Fern. "However, the best type of fitness program for postmenopausal women consists of: flexibility and balance exercises, aerobic weight-bearing exercises, and resistance/strength training."

Flexibility exercises are designed for stretching out muscles and mobilizing joints.

Aerobic weight-bearing exercises, which are excellent for your cardiovascular system, include brisk walking, jogging, stair climbing, jumping rope, tennis, and dancing. These exercises, which are performed against the force of gravity, help increase bone density. Biking and swimming are also good forms of cardiovascular exercise but not as beneficial for your bones.

Resistance and strength training include free weights and resistance bands. Strength training machines are an essential element for increasing bone density.

"Did you know," asked Fern, "that you not only can prevent shrinking as you age, but you can actually increase your height by maintaining good habits?" Before anyone had an opportunity to respond, she quickly cited herself as an example.

"I have actually grown one and a half inches over the past five years, and I'm forty-six!" Standing proudly and with good posture, Fern made a positive statement by her appearance alone. "That's true! If you stand erect without slouching, maintain a daily exercise routine, and watch your diet plus taking supplementary vitamins and calcium, you, too, can preserve your bones so you won't shrink and may even appear taller, as I do.

"The average woman over the age of forty-three," she continued, "loses about 1 percent of her height annually. You might not think that this sounds like much, but it does explain why a young woman of 5'6" may only measure 5'3" tall by the time she reaches eighty.

"In conclusion," said Fern, "I want to point out that shrinkage is due to several factors: first, muscle atrophy; second, vertebral fractures or wedging fractures of the vertebrae; third, disk deterioration; and fourth, poor posture.

"Although a certain amount of shrinkage may be unavoidable for all of us, we can help ourselves by standing tall. Place your feet six inches apart, tuck in your buttocks, suck in your stomach, pull

Postural Changes Associated with Spinal Osteoporosis Without Hormonal Therapy

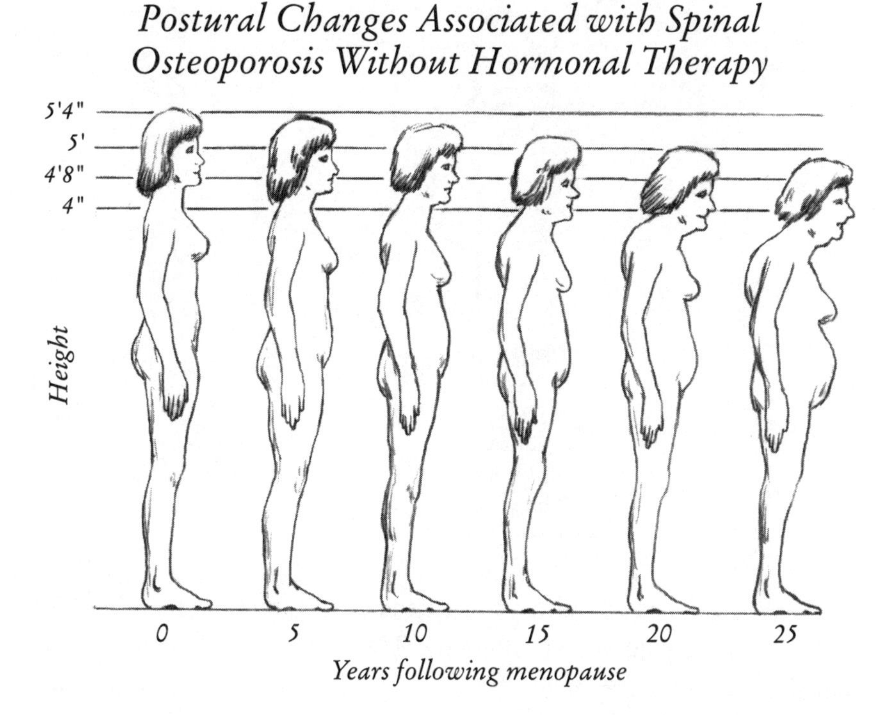

back and down your shoulders, lift up your ears without raising your chin, and, you will look not only self-confident and poised but taller."

So ended our session on fitness. As a final note here, the trend today is to give long-term estrogen replacement therapy for the purpose of preventing osteoporosis and heart disease, conditions that are increasingly likely to develop in women after menopause. Prior to the onset of menopause, large amounts of estrogen are secreted from the ovaries, and smaller amounts from the adrenal glands. Only those women in their late sixties and beyond who show no signs of osteoporosis or heart disease are exempt from needing ERT.

Although much controversy remains on the subject of ERT, it appears the benefits outweigh the risks. A study is presently under way to determine who will benefit the most from ERT. Data from this study will be released from the Women's Health Initiative, a large-scale government-sponsored investigation, though not until 2007.[12]

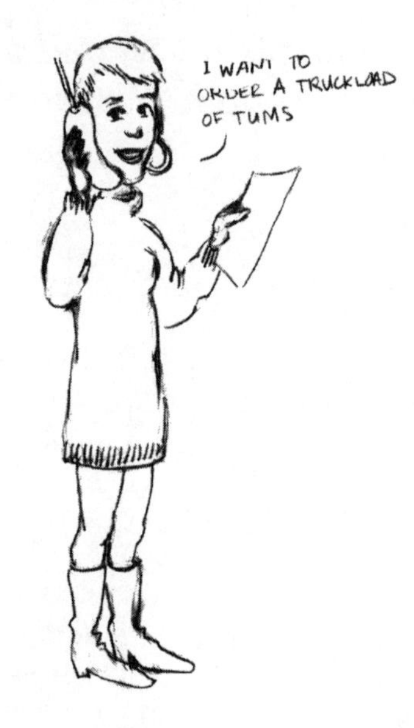

MY OWN experience with a bone density test, after hearing Fern's discussion, proved very interesting. The Osteoporosis Prevention and Research Center at Highland Park Hospital is a state-of-the-art facility dedicated to educating the public about osteoporosis, its prevention and treatment, while providing the most comprehensive diagnosis of the disease.

I was ushered into an examining room by a specially trained nurse clinician who first measured my height, then asked routine questions relating to my family history and personal background that would help in determining my own susceptibility.

This noninvasive test is both safe and painless, lasting only a few minutes as you lie comfortably on a table and the scanner measures bone density of your hip and spine. Afterwards, you are given a complete evaluation as well as suggestions on how to improve your diet and the possibility of vitamin supplements. Your own physician receives a full report.

Criteria for diagnosing osteoporosis range from normal bone density to severe osteoporosis, the middle ranges known as *osteopenia*. I fell into this middle range, having lost 25 percent of my bone density since age thirty, when peak bone mass is reached. Doctors use the percentage of bone lost since age thirty as an indicator of your risk for a fracture. If, for example, at age fifty I had only lost 10 percent of my bone mass, then I would have expected to have a lifetime fracture risk of 30 percent. A 20 percent loss would have doubled my risk; and had it been as high as 30 percent, it would have doubled again, reaching 120 percent. Therefore, my risk factor puts me into the 100 percentile range of possible fractures during my own lifetime. Indeed, one year after I took this test I fractured my foot—swimming! I hit my foot against the side of the pool doing laps.

SESSION 5: DIANNA BOLEN

I began the next session by welcoming my coauthor Dianna Bolen, who has an independent psychotherapy practice: "Dianna does family therapy, individual therapy, marital counseling, and sex therapy. Although Dianna and I did not discuss the details of tonight's talk, I would imagine that it would be something like: 'Sex can be just as fulfilling *after* surgery as before.'"

"Tonight I'm going to talk about a journey," began Dianna. "If you have had pelvic surgery or are facing the prospect of such a surgery, you are embarking on a very personal journey, a journey with a course that is unknown. You will also have many decisions to make along your journey, although not everything will be within your control.

"Your journey can begin to go in one direction, and then another. It can be positive or negative, joyful or tragic, or it can be all of these things. Along this journey you will face challenges that could not have been predicted, as well as some challenges that you can. Your health will be compromised; your body will be irrevocably altered. As a result you may have to change; you may be compelled to reinvent how you think about yourself—who you are, and what is important.

"It is in the context of your personal journey that I want to address your sexual being—your sex life. Your sex life is inextricably interwoven with your personality and your relationships.

"I am here to talk about sex and to get you to think about sex. You may snicker or blush and I'm likely to lapse into a double entendre, here and there, but we're still going to get this sex topic out in the open. So, let's begin!

"Before beginning any journey it's important to know three things: (1) where you are starting from, (2) what kind of a traveler you are, and (3) where you want to go? It is very similar when we talk about your sexual functioning. It also helps to know how you got to be the sexual person you are today, your sexual experiences leading up to this point and the type of sexual experiences you would like to experience in the future.

"It has been my experience that everyone has a 'sexual self-image' that began when each one of us was very young and was shaped by thoughts and events along the way. Each woman's sexual self-image is unique to her. That is because your sexuality is a very personal thing.

"Now, I want to assure you right at the start that even though the topic is sex, you will not be asked to reveal any personal sexual information. Most people don't talk about their sexuality with just anyone, so you won't be asked to do that here. However, I do need you to spend some time thinking about yourself and how you've been sexually, throughout your lifetime. This will give you important background information that will help you see your posthysterectomy sexual self-image in its proper context. For the most part you can expect that your sexual self-image will not be damaged by having had a hysterectomy. However, you may be forced to reevaluate your beliefs about yourself and choose to make some lifestyle adjustments.

"OK, let's talk about sex! Sexual activity is not a priority for some women, it is something they do infrequently or because they assume it's what is required to please their partner. For others it becomes an obsession; for another group, a recreation; and I could go on and on. But right now our goal is to find out what your sexuality has been like for you. So, let's continue.

"Now, please sit back, relax, and imagine; think about your very first sexual feeling. Can you remember how that first sexual feeling came to be? What did you feel? Remember that feeling if you can. What was your response to that new feeling? Please take time to really remember, then write down two or three words that describe your reaction to your first sexual feeling.

"Can you recall a time when you felt desire? How was it to have that feeling? Write down one word that describes your reaction to feeling desire.

"Who was your first sexual partner? Were you a willing participant? What kind of an experience was that? Write down two or three words that describe your first sexual experience.

"When and how did you learn about orgasms? What was that like? (Not all women experience orgasms, but we all know about them.) How important is it to you that you have orgasms? How has your ability to have an orgasm changed (or not changed) over your life, prior to hysterectomy? Write down the answer to this last question.

"What about sexual or romantic fantasies? Most people imagine being with someone or doing things that may not in reality actually ever happen. Some people use fantasies to help provide comfort when their needs cannot be satisfied. Do you get pleasure or satisfaction from your imagination? Write down the kind of fantasies you have (i.e., sexual, romantic, none). No need to write out your specific fantasy.

"Have you ever been having sex and discovered that you really weren't paying attention to what was going on with your partner, as if your mind were somewhere else? Is it important to keep focused on the activity at hand? Write down what helps you keep your mind on sex.

"Do you find yourself not having enough energy for sex? Do you postpone sex in favor of other activities? Write down how your energy for sex, prior to hysterectomy, has changed over the years, if it has.

"Have you ever been swept away with passion, been so aroused that you ached, or delayed sexual gratification so that feelings could become more intense? Write down the word that comes to mind when you think about these experiences.

"What do you think about wearing sexy undergarments? Visiting a sex toy store? Using a vibrator? Write down if you ever would indulge in these activities, and what would make you do any of the above with your partner.

"Now that you have spent some time thinking about sex, you may have an emotional reaction to the process and/or a physical reaction. Take a moment and identify what you are feeling. Write down the feeling.

"Take a breath and exhale slowly. Now look at your list of words. Are they mostly positive, neutral, negative? What does your list of words say about you? Has there been any noticeable change in your sex drive prior to hysterectomy?

"Sexual activity and sensuality are something people do to varying degrees, with differing levels of interest and energy. Even though the differences are many, the following rule of thumb generally applies. The quality of your sexual, and sensual, relationship is determined by the quality of your relationship as a whole. Loving relationships usually result in loving sex; detached relationships usually result in detached sex. A fulfilling relationship begets fulfilling sex.

"When people talk about sex, they may be referring to any number of activities, some of which do not include intercourse or orgasm. I'm using the word *sex* to describe a wide range of activities which involve physical, sensual pleasure.

"Sexual and sensual functioning involve a greater area than just the female genitalia. It involves your skin, your lips, your eyes, and your mind! But for starters, let's review the parts of the female genital anatomy. These include: *vulva,* the visible part of the female anatomical structure; *clitoris,* the erogenous erectile tissue located above the opening of the vagina (the female counterpart of the penis); *labia,* the lips of the female genitalia on either side of the entrance to the vagina; *vagina,* the female mucous membrane canal leading from the vulva to the cervix of the uterus, the canal in which copulation takes place. For some women, there is an area of heightened sensitivity at the frontal portion of the vagina, about two inches inside. Other women report that their most sensitive

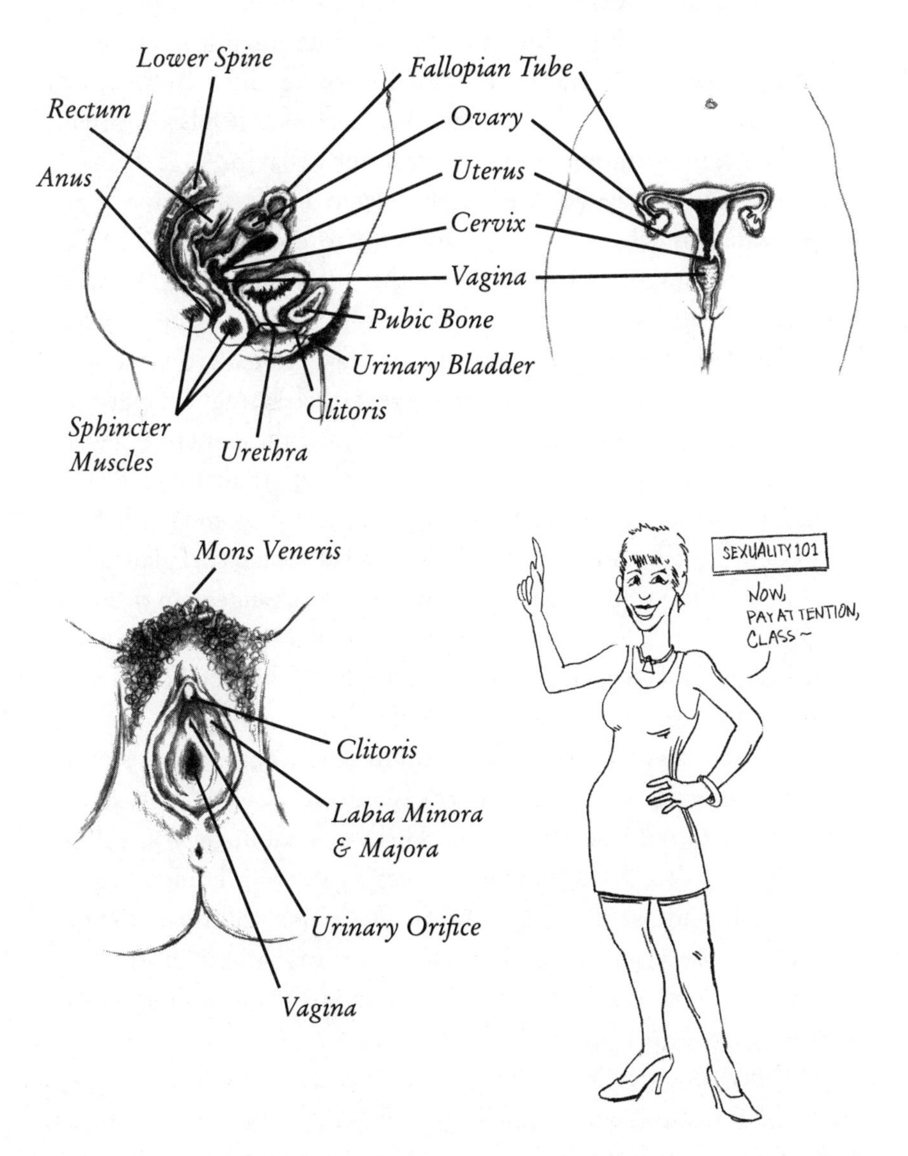

area is the tip of the cervix. Most women, however, feel that the clitoris is the most highly sensitive and erotic area. Remember, though, that you are not 'most women'; your erotic areas are unique to you. It is your responsibility to know and to communicate the ways in which you like to receive pleasure.

"Sexual behavior is affected by your hormone level, and hormone levels are affected by your behavior. Certain behaviors, like taking supplements, getting enough rest, minimizing stress, exercising, masturbating, and other sexually stimulating activities, can affect hormone levels. As we age, our hormone levels drop, and that change in hormone level can affect our behavior.

"Hormones/behavior are closely related and feed upon one another, which is why it is very important to consider taking HRT after pelvic surgery. Testosterone, the male hormone, is what supplies us with sexual motivation and the ability to enjoy sexual fantasies. Some premenopausal women take testosterone supplements just to increase their sex drive. Nevertheless, regular, vigorous exercise may also result in a modest increase in testosterone levels. Our sexual behavior can also stimulate our body to increase its hormonal levels because even after a hysterectomy women still have ways of producing hormones. One way is via the adrenal glands.

"In addition to decreased hormone levels, changes can occur to your genitals from lack of blood flow to that area. Increased blood flow brings vital oxygen and other nutrients to your cells, allowing them to function properly. Your genitals are made up of cells just like all other parts of your body. Stimulation to orgasm or simple gentle massaging of the genital area is a good way to increase the flow of blood to the genital region. This can be done by yourself or with the help of a partner. When massaging or stimulating the genital area, it is advisable to use a lubricant, which will make the experience more enjoyable. The availability of natural lubrication decreases as you age, just like your skin and nails lose moisture as you age.

"Many people (particularly men) equate the presence of natural lubrication with sexual arousal. This is not true. Various factors can contribute to the lack of lubrication, including but not limited to the use of antihistamine medications. Do you think the drying effects of cold or allergy medications are limited to your nose?

"Regardless of the reason, be it a hormonal deficiency or the use of drugs which cause dryness, lack of lubrication should not eliminate one's enjoyment of sex. A variety of lubricants are available on the market; Replens and Astroglide are two I recommend.

"Stay away from Vaseline products," cautioned Dianna. "They don't absorb and are difficult to remove. Vaseline-like products are made from petroleum, which is similar to motor oil. It is slippery (which is good) but cannot be easily removed (which is bad). Ever get motor oil on your clothing? You need plenty of soap and water as well as lots of scrubbing. The sensitive tissues of your genitals and vagina will not respond well to that treatment. Also, petroleum melts latex, the material comprising condoms, which obviously lessens their effectiveness in preventing disease and pregnancy.

"Now, about orgasms," continued Dianna. "Contrary to what you may have heard, pelvic surgery does not eliminate orgasms even though your internal anatomy has been altered. Your experience, however, may be different after surgery. It's also possible that your first postsurgical sexual encounter may fail, if you are measuring your success in terms of having an orgasm. You must keep trying. The ability to achieve orgasm is a skill, like any other, and that skill can be learned, forgotten, and relearned. Even for some animals, mating is a learned skill.

"Also, women can achieve orgasm in more than one way. Women have reported to experiencing orgasms through fantasy alone, stimulation of the nipples, repeated squeezing together of the thighs, anal penetration, direct clitoral stimulation, and intercourse. Most women have never experienced deep uterine orgasms, but orgasm by other means, usually stimulation to the clitoris. The point here is that if one or more of your sexual parts has been removed, you still retain a range of options for sexual and sensual pleasure. Your mind retains a kinesthetic, or 'feeling,' memory of your body as it was prior to having been compromised. You may have heard that war veterans, those who have lost limbs, report that they can still feel sensations in those missing parts. We have a long way to go before understanding why.

"I won't deny that sex after surgery can be different, but I *will* argue with anyone who believes that 'good' sex cannot be achieved after hysterectomy. Many woman experience no difference in sex after a hysterectomy. Some say sex is better.

"Since sex usually happens with a partner, I want to address partner issues here. First of all, it is likely that your partner has been disturbed by your surgery. Although I'm going to speak about heterosexual relationships here, the same would hold true for lesbian partners. Your partner cannot see inside you, so he can only imagine what has changed, what is different. Your partner has probably seen the scar and has had to deal with his response to seeing it. It's OK to talk about how it is for you to have a scar. He probably is also afraid to hurt you, to cause you additional pain. I have treated men who had temporarily lost their ability to get an erection because of the fear of causing their partner pain. But, the erection had to do with his fears, not the woman's desirability.

"Depending on your partner's degree of emotional maturity and his ability to handle the stresses associated with your surgery, interpersonal problems could develop. Sometimes these problems have actually been there all along, lying dormant under the surface of the relationship. The additional stress of the surgery brings them to the surface.

"Partners may become insecure or impatient because they don't understand the changes which have taken place. Learning how to talk openly with your partner about this and teaching your partner how to give you pleasure will be helpful to you both. Normally, if you have not been able to communicate openly about sex prior to the surgery, it won't be any easier now. Nancy said the opposite in her story. Sometimes the aftermath of surgery provides the extra initiative to take some risks and engage in new behaviors. Open communication is risky, but healthy! Emotional and physical intimacy work together to make a richly satisfying sexual relationship.

"Because it's hard to predict what it will be like to have sex after surgery, some people may try to avoid it for as long as possible. Both men and women will come up with a myriad of excuses: 'I'm too tired,' 'I don't feel well,' 'The kids may still be awake,' 'I'm afraid it might hurt,' 'I just had my hair done,' 'My nails are wet,' 'I have work to do,' 'I'm watching a good movie'—to name just a few. However, if you stop making excuses and begin to physically please each other, the outcome is usually positive. As you gain experience, you will also gain confidence. Nondemanding physical contact is a wonderful place to start. There is much to be said for simple hugging and holding, stroking and snuggling before falling asleep in each other's arms.

"Good sexual relations will be further enhanced after pelvic surgery by strengthening the pubococcygeal (PC) muscles, otherwise known as Kegel muscles. These muscles were named after Dr. Arnold Kegel, who developed a system of exercises in the late 1940s. The Kegels, located in the genital region, extend from the bladder to the vagina and anus. In relearning how to properly use them, you can do simple daily exercises by contracting these muscles and then releasing them.

> *"Physically healthy people, those who follow a regular daily exercise routine, are also better fit sexually. Exercise not only improves muscle tone but also increases a person's level of testosterone, which in turn affects the libido."*

"You can locate the Kegel muscles by voluntary interruption of the urinary stream, but caution should be observed; frequent interruption of the urinary stream can be harmful to the bladder. Kegel muscles are useful for jump-starting an orgasm, like the engine of a car is jump-started with booster cables. Remember, unused muscles will atrophy—use them or lose them!

"Physically healthy people, those who follow a regular daily exercise routine, are also better fit sexually. Exercise not only improves muscle tone but also increases a person's level of testosterone, which in turn affects the libido.

"In certain situations, not necessarily related to hysterectomy, normal coitus cannot be performed either because of a serious, chronic illness or radical surgery, which may affect either partner. Under these circumstances, a loving relationship can still be maintained by a couple's close contact, and physical intimacy can be enjoyed in different ways."

An example of such intimacy was revealed by Bonnie, a forty-six-year-old woman, married with no children, who had undergone a radical hysterectomy for cervical cancer a year and a half earlier. Her husband, twelve years her senior, had undergone radical surgery plus radiation therapy for prostate cancer the year before.

Bonnie described her marital relations since having had surgery in this way: "We feel closer than ever. I did go through a post-surgical depression for six months but didn't go for help because my husband is strong and supportive. He understood what I was going through because his surgery took away his manhood. Mine robbed me of my womanhood. We can't have sexual relations anymore, but I don't feel lonely. We have a loving relationship and hug and kiss all the time. We're very close."

Then Dianna opened the discussion period. Judy was the first of the group to respond.

"Speaking about intercourse," began Judy, "oral sex should not be discounted. Many women prefer oral sex."

"Yes, I agree wholeheartedly!" replied Dianna. "Oral sex is enjoyed by many women, both the giving and the receiving. By some women it is the preferred sexual activity, although many women are hesitant to clearly state their preference for oral sex. If you want oral sex, ask for it. If you want to give oral sex, go for it."

Dianna waited for additional questions; no one ventured.

"What about pain after surgery?" asked Dianna, attempting to stimulate a discussion. "Is it temporary or permanent? How have you dealt with the short-term or in some cases long-term discomfort associated with your surgery? You know, in some cases the length of the vagina is shortened during surgery, and both the woman *and* her partner must adapt to these changes."

Dianna probed further. "What about anger?"

Dead silence.

"Come on, gals," I urged. "If we're honest with ourselves, *all* of us had to have experienced at least moments of anger if not a full-blown case of postsurgical depression. I cried my eyes out for at least ten minutes one night in the hospital. It's normal!"

"In my own practice," said Dr. Metres, "I have found that women who have been sexually abused seem most affected by a hysterectomy because of its very invasiveness."

"When a person has experienced sexual trauma, particularly if it has been repeated trauma over a period of months or years," Dianna added, "she tends to be more vulnerable to being retraumatized by an invasive procedure like hysterectomy. In some cases, there can even be a psychotic break for a brief period of time, when the patient may actually *mentally* cease to function.

"A hysterectomy, and the loss of those very personal body parts, holds unique meaning for each woman who experiences it. Recently, I read an article in which three women reported having been robbed of their creativity after having undergone hysterectomies during their childbearing years."

"Depending on one's moral or religious background," Mary interjected, "a hysterectomy can lead to enormous sexual freedom. As a Catholic, I was brought up to believe that any form of birth control was a sin. For over twenty-five years I was surrounded by nuns. But the church hasn't banned sex following a hysterectomy, and that's the greatest birth control of all! For the first time I now feel totally unburdened and can enjoy being just plain sexual."

"Even from a secular standpoint," I replied, "a hysterectomy gives women complete sexual freedom without the fear of pregnancy."

"Yes," added Ann, "and it's nice to enjoy being empty nesters. Getting back together and focusing upon each other makes this time of life very special. I don't grieve for my lost organs. In fact, a couple weeks ago I had an ultrasound taken, and after a few minutes I said to the technician, 'You aren't finished already, are you?' But, to my surprise, she replied, 'Why, yes—there's not much left to scan.' Nor was that the first time someone poked fun about my being barren. But I don't care. It's not important."

"It has been my experience," commented Dianna, "that many women actually report an improvement in their quality of life after surgery. They feel less fatigue, and some report a higher level of energy."

"I had surgery very recently," replied Mary. "It's true that you do need to communicate with your partner because things may be different after surgery. If you have someone who can rise to the occasion. . . . ," Her words trailed off as the room, once again, swelled with uncontrollable laughter at Mary's innocent play on words.

"True!" replied Dianna, delighting in the humor just created by Mary's last remark. "Men don't know enough about hysterectomies, but they're teachable."

"Men," fired Judy, defensively, "go through their own hell with prostate even though some don't even seem to understand what prostate's all about." Dr. Metres jumped in to defend men.

"That's because men are far more frightened about prostate and testicular cancer," he said. "There's an unwillingness among men to communicate these feelings with other men. That's a big problem."

Dianna closed the session by summarizing the discussion.

"The female sexual response can be affected by (1) sexual drive and libido (hormonal); (2) organic aspects (tissue conditions, muscles, lubrication); (3) skill and learning (sensual joy leading to orgasm—'practice makes perfect'); (4) receptivity (one's mental condition, ability to be a sexual person); (5) relational (two people feeling comfortable, trust and love).

"In each of these five areas you can make choices that will result in enhancing your sexual and sensual functioning, if that is what you want. Your sex life is your choice."

THE WOMEN'S workshop had concluded, and it felt as if a huge weight had been lifted from my shoulders. Yet this was really not an ending, only another beginning.

REFLECTIONS

WRITING THIS book has been an immensely interesting, educating, and fulfilling experience. I am particularly grateful to the women who gave of their time to share their personal stories with me. I think we have learned from all of them. For me personally, their strength has given me strength, and their courage has inspired me to be more honest and open about my own situation.

When I finished what I thought would be the last sentence of this book, I casually glanced up at the calendar. The date was Wednesday, September 3, 1997—exactly one year to the day of my surgery. It had occurred to me that while, perhaps, my story had been brought to closure, other women's stories were just beginning.

Dianna Bolen and I planned a meeting for Saturday when she would have her first peek at the completed work. Unfortunately, I had been remiss. I had neglected to phone Dianna earlier because of my self-absorption with writing the manuscript even though she had done all the scientific analysis on the questionnaires.

In reflecting on the events of that year, I had come to realize more clearly than ever the significance of those events. Not only had it been a year of physical healing, but, more important, it had been a year of personal growth. I feel stronger and healthier now than ever before, and I have also come to terms with many unresolved issues.

Toward the end of this project, as days merged with sleepless nights as I sat at my computer, I was still struggling to fit all the puzzle pieces together. Then, as if someone had entered the room and suddenly snapped on the lights, my vision was instantly restored. All at once I understood what my experience had taught me, and I could see the personal growth that had come from moving through this life challenge. I also knew what my message to other women facing similar challenges would be:

Responsibility: Every one of us should be accountable to ourselves rather than relying on the judgment of others. For example, when confronted with a serious issue that affects our very health and well-being, we first need to understand the nature of the problem rather than being blindly dependent on other people—even doctors! Do your homework, become informed, and then you will be prepared to discuss your situation with your doctor more intelligently. Remember: the ultimate responsibility regarding surgery rests in your hands; it is *your* body.

Self-empowerment: Developing the art of self-empowerment can be invaluable to each and every woman. My way of feeling empowered was to study and plan ahead, thereby taking control of my own situation wherever I could.

Carol, one of the woman interviewed who had survived uterine cancer, dealt pragmatically with her "no-option" situation with a positive attitude. After accepting surgery as her only alternative, she assumed responsibility for herself by becoming informed. Carol was then in a position to help in the decision-making process regarding the actual procedure. Although surgery was mandatory, she had some control over the type of incision as well as the possibility of retaining her ovaries. She even arranged for an endocrinologist to be present during the operation just in case her ovaries needed to be removed. In the final analysis, Carol's ovaries were spared.

Humor: Humor not only helps ease your own pain but also makes those people around you feel more relaxed and comfortable. You can appreciate the moment. Being able to poke fun at ourselves not only releases tension but also provides us with an opportunity to step back and take a fresh look at our situation. A new perspective can make all the difference. Furthermore, laughter has been proven to boost the immune system and lower blood pressure. A good belly laugh is good medicine.

From reading the examples in this book, you can see the importance of taking responsibility into your own hands. You should also have a clear understanding of the concept of empowerment, and humor cannot be overly stressed.

Like most people, I had experienced a real dread of surgery. Nevertheless, with competent doctors and a well-equipped, well-staffed hospital, surgery of this type is no longer a major threat. People seldom die from anesthesia, and surgery is usually performed *only* when absolutely necessary.

The fears of being "castrated" and losing my feminine identity have also been reconciled. Both were gross misconceptions! Body parts can be surgically removed, but no operation can rob a woman of her womanhood. A woman is just as much a woman, with or without her reproductive system.

We all have our strengths and weaknesses, and we all experience loss of one kind or another. But through it all, if we can arrive at true self-acceptance, we will experience the healing necessary for our individual lives. At the end of my year-long "hysterectomy journey," I had come to accept myself and had developed the ability to accept and understand others more fully. The opportunity to be involved with those other women who shared part of their journey with me has greatly enriched my life.

Birth is a beginning
And death a destination.
And life is a journey . . .
From innocence to awareness
And ignorance to knowing;
From foolishness to discretion

And then, perhaps, to wisdom;
From weakness to strength
Or strength to weakness
And, often, back again . . .
From defeat to defeat to defeat
Until, looking backward or ahead,
We see that victory lies
Not at some high place along the way,
But in having made the journey, stage by stage . . .
Birth is a beginning . . .
And life is a journey.[1]

APPENDIX A: STATISTICAL DATA OF RESEARCH QUESTIONNAIRE

NAME (optional)	
SIGNED	43
ANONYMOUS	32
AGE (Unanswered: 8)	
26–30	2
31– 40	8
41– 50	17
51– 60	22
61– 70	13
71– 82	5
MARITAL STATUS (Unanswered: 5)	
Married	56
Single	4
Separated/divorced	8
Widowed	2
DATE OF SURGERY (Unanswered: 4)	
1997–1990	31
1989–1980	20
1979–1970	8
1969–1960	10
1953	1
1939 (at 24 years old)	1

TYPE OF SURGERY (Unanswered: 11)

Vaginal hysterectomy	15
Laparoscopically assisted vaginal hysterectomy	1
Subtotal hysterectomy	7
Total hysterectomy	14
Total hysterectomy with bilateral salpingo-ovariectomy	17
Total hysterectomy with unilateral salpingo-ovariectomy	3
Radical hysterectomy	2
Myomectomy	7

If abdominal surgery, please indicate type of incision:

Vertical	26
Bikini	24

1. Was this *required* or *elective* surgery? Please explain.

Required	56
Elective	16
Uncertain	3

Conditions requiring surgery:

Bleeding	15
Tumors/fibroid	19
Prolapsed uterus	3
Malignancy	6
Precancer	8
Endometriosis	7
Cysts	5
Other	16

2. If surgery was elective, do you feel the decision was justified by the outcome?

Yes	13
No	1
Uncertain	2

3. Did your physician fully inform you of the facts, and did you go for a 2nd/3rd opinion?

Yes	56
No	11
2nd+ opinions	25

4. How did you prepare yourself for surgery mentally and physically?

None	14
Tests	1
Acceptance/good attitude	31
Took time	5
Had fears	4
Felt rushed	6
Spiritual	3
Researched	9
Support	8

5. Did you arrange for a relative or friend to help you at home with meals, housework, and child care after surgery? Please explain.

Husband/boyfriend	17
Mother	12
Father	5
Son/daughter	9
Sister	1
Other family	9
Friend(s)	6
Hired	11

6. Were you aware of the physical changes following hysterectomy? How did you adjust?

Yes	75
No	0
Felt fine	32
Specific +	5

Specific –	14
Hormones	8

7. Did you suffer from postsurgical depression? If so, what happened, and how did you cope? (Unanswered: 4)

Yes	12
No	51
Recovery took time	3
Received or sought support	5

8. Has the quality of your life changed as a result of surgery? Please explain.

Yes +	29
Yes –	9
No	26
Uncertain	11

9. Has surgery affected your sex life? Please explain. (Unanswered: 10)

Improved	18
No	34
Uncertain (too soon)	4
Negative	9

10. Have you experienced marital difficulties since your hysterectomy? (Unanswered: 14)

Yes	3
No	43
N/A	15

11. Have your weight and appetite changed since surgery?

Yes	25
No	35
Uncertain	15

12. Did you begin hormone replacement therapy after surgery? If so, what are you taking? If not, why?

Yes	39
No	32
N/A	4

Types of HRT:

Premarin	21
Estrace	8
Estratest	2
Progesterone	2
Provera	2
Estrogen-ortho est	1
Estrogen cream	2
Estrogen patch	5
Progesterone cream	1

13. Did you have complications from surgery? If so, what kind? (Unanswered: 9)

Yes	6
No	60

14. Would you recommend surgery for others or suggest nonsurgical options? (Unanswered: 9)

Yes	22
Investigate options	12
Uncertain	7
No opinion	25

APPENDIX B: WORKSHOP SURVEY QUESTIONNAIRE*

1. Please evaluate the helpfulness of the workshop series as a whole (from 0, which equals not helpful at all; to 7, which equals extremely helpful): 5.5
2. Please assign a helpfulness rating number (0–7) to each of the sessions:

   Session 1: 4.0
   Session 2: 6.0
   Session 3: 5.0
   Session 4: 6.0
   Session 5: 6.0
3. What might improve the workshop series?

   "Better development of relationships within the group."
   "Begin first session by sitting in a circle, not classroom style, and introducing each other (first name only)."

   "Efforts to protect confidentiality were appropriate and should be continued."

   "If the workshop topic is on a medical/surgical problem, a health care–accredited person should be available to separate fact from fiction."
4. Has your attitude toward pelvic surgery changed since the beginning of the series? If so, how?

   "Has been broadened immensely."

*Please note that the responses to questions 2 through 9 represent a compilation from the material collected. Not all participants chose to respond to every subjective question.

"More accepting of the experience and what it's contributed to personal growth."

"Still troubled with the sexual phase after complete hysterectomy."

"Women need to be more in control."

5. Are there any changes you intend to make or have begun) as a result of this workshop?

   "Keep reading. Keep my eyes and ears open for research articles on this issue."

   "More dedication to exercise."

   "Plan to speak some more with my doctor about problems I'm experiencing."

   "Will continue to make changes in diet, exercise patterns, and posture because of the information on osteoporosis."

6. How would rate the emotional support you had prior to the workshop series? 4.0
7. How do you rate your level of support now? 4.5
8. What future workshops might be helpful?

   "Dealing with empty nests."

   "Dealing with aging, sick parents, and spouse."

   "Therapeutic support group."

9. Other comments and suggestions?

   "Thanks, Nancy, for all the attention, research, publicity, support, and love you gave to keep participants and presenters engaged." Phil Metres, Ph.D.

   "Individuals with an agenda unrelated to the workshop are distracting and, perhaps, need to be channeled elsewhere."

Prepared by
Dianna W. Bolen, Psy.D.
DWB Human Services
Chicago, Illinois

NOTES

CHAPTER 1

1. Stacie E. Geller, Lawton R. Burns, and David J. Brailer, "The Impact of Nonclinical Factors on Practice Variations: The Case of Hysterectomies," *Health Services Research,* February 1996, 729.
2. Adelaide Haas and Susan L. Puretz, *The Woman's Guide to Hysterectomy* (Berkeley, CA: Celestial Arts, 1995), 65.
3. Ibid., 39.
4. Ibid., 64.
5. "Hysterectomy and Its Alternatives: One Step Toward Assessing the Options," *HealthFacts* 19, no. 180 (May 1994), 3.
6. Alan E. Nourse, *The Ladies' Home Journal Family Medical Guide* (New York: Harper & Row, 1973), 755–757.
7. Haas and Puretz, *Woman's Guide to Hysterectomy,* 78–79, 82.

CHAPTER 2

1. Nelson H. Stringer, *Uterine Fibroids: What Every Woman Needs to Know* (Glenview, IL: Physicians and Scientists, 1996), 9–12, 19–20.
2. Judith Sachs, *What Women Can Do About Chronic Endometriosis* (New York: Dell, 1991), 5.

CHAPTER 3

1. Judith Reichman, *"I'm Too Young to Get Old"* (New York: Times Books, 1996), 199–200.

CHAPTER 4

1. David A. Grimes, "Primary Prevention of Ovarian Cancer," *Journal of the American Medical Association,* 270 no. 23 (December 15, 1993), 2855.
2. Karen J. Carlson, Stephanie A. Eisenstat, and Terra Ziporyn, *The Harvard Guide to Women's Health* (Cambridge, MA: Harvard University Press, 1966), 351–352.
3. Adelaide Haas and Susan L. Puretz, *The Woman's Guide to Hysterectomy* (Berkeley, CA: Celestial Arts, 1995), 107.
4. Paula Dranov, "When the Diagnosis Is Fibroids: New Treatments Will Prevent Hysterectomy for Millions of Women," *American Health* 12, no. 7 (September 1993), 68.
5. David A. Grimes, "Shifting Indications for Hysterectomy: Nature, Nurture, or Neither?" *Lancet* (December 17, 1994), 1652.

CHAPTER 6

1. Nancy Rosenfeld, *Unfinished Journey: "From Tyranny to Freedom"* (Lanham, MD: University Press of America, 1993); and Yuri Tarnopolsky, *Memoirs of 1984* (Lanham, MD: University Press of America, 1993).
2. Winnifred B. Cutler, *Hysterectomy: Before and After* (New York: HarperPerennial, 1990), 155–156.
3. Ibid., 170–171.
4. Adelaide Haas and Susan L. Puretz, *The Woman's Guide to Hysterectomy* (Berkeley, CA: Celestial Arts, 1995), 107.

CHAPTER 7

1. Dr. Lee Berk, professor of pathology and laboratory medicine at Loma Linda University in California, and Dr. Stanley Tan, Loma Linda University, presented these data at the sixth annual meeting of the American Association for Therapeutic Humor in Orlando, Florida, November 1996.
2. Winnifred B. Cutler, *Hysterectomy: Before and After* (New York: HarperPerennial, 1990), 313–318.

CHAPTER 8

1. Karen J. Carlson, Stephanie A. Eisenstat and Terra Ziporyn, *The Harvard Guide to Women's Health* (Cambridge, MA: Harvard University Press, 1966), 130.
2. L. Helstrom, "Sexuality After Hysterectomy: A Model Based on Quantitative and Qualitative Analysis of 104 Women Before and After Subtotal Hysterectomy," *Journal of Psychosomatic Obstetrics and Gynecology* 15, no. 4 (December 1994), 219–229.

CHAPTER 9

1. Karen J. Carlson, Stephanie A. Eisenstat and Terra Ziporyn, *The Harvard Guide to Women's Health* (Cambridge, MA: Harvard University Press, 1966), 525–526.
2. Ibid., 223.
3. Ibid., 328.

CHAPTER 10

1. Judith Reichman, *"I'm Too Young to Get Old"* (New York: Times Books, 1996), 114–118.
2. Christine Northrup, *Women's Bodies, Women's Wisdom* (New York: Bantam, 1995), 185–186, 587–624.

CHAPTER 13

1. Winnifred B. Cutler, *Hysterectomy: Before and After* (New York: HarperPerennial, 1990), 27–28, 36–37, 116–117, 122–128, 142–143, 147, 191–193, 205–207, 216–222, 273–274.
2. Adelaide Haas and Susan L. Puretz, *The Woman's Guide to Hysterectomy* (Berkeley, CA: Celestial Arts, 1995), 20.
3. Cutler, *Hysterectomy: Before and After*, 130–144.
4. Ibid., 83–84.
5. Karen J. Carlson, Stephanie A. Eisenstat and Terra Ziporyn, *The Harvard Guide to Women's Health* (Cambridge, MA: Harvard University Press, 1966), 630.
6. Haas and Puretz, *Woman's Guide to Hysterectomy*, 78.

7. Cutler, *Hysterectomy: Before and After*, 133–135.
8. Judith Reichman, *"I'm Too Young to Get Old"* (New York: Times Books, 1996), 256–278.
9. Ibid., 135–136, 164.
10. Ibid., 164.
11. Carlson, Eisenstat, and Ziporyn, *Harvard Guide to Women's Health*, 382.
12. Ibid., 234–237.

REFLECTIONS

1. Excerpts from Rabbi Alvin I. Fine's poem are copyright by the Central Conference of American Rabbis and are reproduced with permission.

GLOSSARY

acupuncture—The practice of inserting fine needles into the body to alleviate pain and symptoms.

AIDS—Acquired immune deficiency syndrome, a fatal condition caused by the HTLV-III/LAV virus. The virus destroys T-cell lymphocytes that are essential in protecting the body against infections.

alternative medicine—A holistic approach to curing disease that considers the total person, body and soul.

anesthesia—Loss of sensation, usually produced to permit a painless surgical procedure.

- **caudal**—The injection of an anesthetic agent, such as Novocain, into the lower caudal (spinal) canal near the end of the vertebral column.
- **dissociative**—An anesthesia that doesn't cause complete unconsciousness.
- **endotracheal**—General anesthesia administered through a tube and placed through the mouth or nose, directly into the trachea (windpipe).
- **epidural**—Produced by the injection of an anesthetic agent, such as Novocain, into the space just outside the spinal canal.
- **field block**—A local anesthesia applied directly to the area to be operated on.
- **general**—Any anesthesia associated with loss of consciousness.
- **hypotensive**—An anesthesia given when the blood pressure has been purposely lowered to cut down on operative blood loss.
- **hypothermic**—An anesthesia given when the body temperature has been purposely lowered.
- **inhalation**—Anesthesia produced through the inhalation of gases or vapors.
- **intravenous**—The injection of an anesthetic agent, such as Pentothal, into a vein.

peripheral—Loss of sensation in the nerves of the skin.

regional—Anesthesia restricted to a part of the body.

saddle block—Spinal anesthesia given so as to affect only the genital region, buttocks, and thighs.

spinal—That produced by the injection of an anesthetic agent, such as Novocain, directly into the spinal fluid within the spinal canal.

topical—Application of an anesthetic agent on a body surface, as with a spray or cotton swab.

anesthesiologist—A physician who specializes in the administration of anesthesia.

anus—The outlet of the gastrointestinal tract; the final one or one and one-half inches of the rectum.

arterial embolization—A procedure to shrink fibroids in which the surgeon inserts a catheter into an artery in the woman's leg and moves the catheter within the artery up to where the artery supplies the fibroid. At this supply point a foam or propylvinyl alcohol is injected into the artery to block the blood flow.

autologous blood donation—Donation of one's own blood, kept available for your own use if needed during surgery.

benign—A noncancerous condition; nonmalignant.

beta carotene—A naturally occurring pigment with immunity-enhancing properties present in yellow, orange, and leafy, dark green vegetables.

bikini cut—See *Pfannestiel incision.*

biopsy—The surgical removal of tissue to determine the exact diagnosis. Tumors are often submitted to biopsy while the patient is on the operating table.

breakthrough bleeding—Spotting or irregularly occurring endometrial discharges not associated with menstruation.

cancer—A malignant tumor of any type.

carcinogenic—Producing or causing cancer.

carcinoma—Cancer derived from lining cells of organs. It can occur in almost any structure of the body.

cardiovascular disease—A disease relating to the heart and blood vessels, or vascular system.

castration—Removal of the male testicles; see also *oopherectomy.*

catheter—A rubber, plastic, or glass tube inserted into the bladder to withdraw urine.

catheterization—Withdrawal of urine from the bladder by passage of a tube.

CAT scan—The simultaneous taking of many X-rays from many angles, giving a highly defined set of pictures of an organ or organs; also known as *computerized axial tomography.*

CBC—Stands for *complete blood count.*

cervix—The entrance and lower portion of the uterus.

cesarean—Also *C-section;* the delivery of a child through a cut in the abdomen.

chemotherapy—Treatment of infection or tumors through the use of chemical agents.

cholesterol—A chemical component of animal oils and fats. Excessive amounts are deposited in blood vessels and may be a factor in the causation of hardening of the arteries (arteriosclerosis).

chronic—Of long duration; not acute.

climax—Orgasm; a series of strong, involuntary contractions of the muscles of the genitalia experienced as pleasurable.

clitoris—Part of the external female genitals, containing erectile tissue and located above the opening that leads from the bladder. The penis is the male counterpart of the clitoris.

coitus—Sexual intercourse.

complete hysterectomy—See *total hysterectomy.*

contraindication—A medical term used to highlight effects that are at cross purposes to each other (e.g., birth control pills are contraindicated for women with fibroid tumors because they are likely to cause an increase in the rate of fibroid growth).

corpus luteum—A small yellowish area in an ovary found at the site where an egg has formed and burst from the gland.

cyst—A sac containing fluid, blood, sweat gland secretions, and so forth.

D&C—See *dilation and curettage.*

dilation and curettage—Also known as D&C, a method of opening (dilating) the cervix and scraping tissue from the endometrium (with a curette) for diagnostic or treatment purposes.

ectopic pregnancy—Development of the embryo outside of the uterus.

EKG—See *electrocardiogram.*

electrocardiogram—A test that records the electrical impulses of the heart. These tracings can detect heart abnormalities and disease.

endometriosis—The presence of cells that line the uterus in unusual places, such as in the bladder or intestinal wall. This condition can cause painful menstruation and sterility.

endometrium—The mucous membrane lining the uterine cavity.

erogenous zone—An area that, when stimulated, arouses sexual feelings.

ERT—See *estrogen replacement therapy.*

estrogen replacement therapy (ERT)—The use of estrogen postmenopausally to help prevent cardiovascular disease and osteoporosis, relief from menopausal symptoms as well as positive effects on skin and mucous membranes.

fallopian tubes—The uterine tubes, one on either side of the uterus; the passageways through which the egg passes from the ovary to the uterus.

fibroids—Benign (noncancerous) tumors composed of fibrous and fat tissue, stemming from the smooth muscle of the uterus.

flushes—See *hot flashes.*

gamete intrafallopian transfer (GIFT)—An assisted reproduction technique; the eggs and sperm are placed into the fallopian tubes via laparoscopy before fertilization has occurred.

gestational surrogacy—A woman, whose uterus is damaged or missing, has her own eggs fertilized with her partner's sperm and implanted into the womb of another woman who becomes the surrogate.

GIFT—See *gamete intrafallopian transfer.*

gonadotropin-releasing hormones (GnRH)—Hormones used as a temporary measure to shrink the size of fibroids before surgical removal.

gonads—The sex glands; the ovaries or testicles.

Grafenberg area—Also G-spot; an area on the front portion of the vagina that is supposed to be especially sensitive to stimulation. The existence and importance of a G-spot are controversial.

gynecologist—A physician specializing in diseases of women, especially those of the reproductive organs.

gynecology—That branch of medicine dealing with female anatomy, physiology, health, and, specifically, the reproductive organs.

health maintenance organization (HMO)—An organization that oversees the delivery of medical services by a limited group of physicians and hospitals.

herbal medicine—The use of balms and medications prepared from flowers, leaves, and other parts of plants.

high-density lipoproteins (HDLs)—Protein molecules that carry cholesterol from the blood to the liver.

HMO—See *health maintenance organization.*

holistic medicine—A system of total patient care that takes into consideration physical, spiritual, and emotional factors as well as the social and economic aspects in the maintenance of health and the treatment of illness.

homeopathy—A botanical alternative of medicine that treats disease with small doses of the same substance that caused it.

hormone—A chemical produced by a gland, secreted into the bloodstream, and affecting the function of distant cells or organs.

hormone replacement therapy (HRT)—A general term used for any hormonal treatment (i.e., estrogen replacement with or without progesterone).

hot flashes—A sudden increase in body temperature, often followed by profuse perspiration, associated with menopause in some women.

HRT—See *hormone replacement therapy.*

hymen—A thin membrane covering the entrance to the vagina.

hyperplasia—Overactive cells that can become cancerous.

hypertension—High blood pressure.

hysterectomy—Surgical removal of the uterus.

hysterectomy with bilateral salpingo-oopherectomy—Surgical removal of the uterus, ovaries, and fallopian tubes.

incontinence—Involuntary voiding or involuntary passage of stool or urine.

in vitro fertilization (IVF)—An assisted reproduction technique in which an egg is taken from a woman's ovary, fertilized by a man's sperm in a laboratory, and then transplanted into the mother's womb. Also known as *laboratory fertilization.* IVF is a good choice for women who have damaged or blocked fallopian tubes.

isometric—Of equal proportions.

IVF—See *in vitro fertilization.*

Kegel exercises—Exercises used to strengthen genital muscles.

keloid—A knotty overgrowth of a scar, sometimes forming after surgery.

labia—Lips of the female genitalia on either side of the vagina.

laparoscope—An instrument used for viewing the interior of the abdomen.

laparoscopic hysterectomy—A procedure for removal of the uterus with the aid of the laparoscope.

laparoscopy—The examination of the abdominal cavity by insertion of a lighted, hollow metal instrument.

laser—*L*ight *a*mplification by *s*timulated *e*missions of *r*adiation; the use of focused light in surgical procedures that produces the most intense heat, capable of destroying tumor masses when aimed in their direction.

LDLs—See *low-density lipoproteins.*

libido—Sexual desire and sex drive.

low-density lipoproteins (LDLs)—Protein molecules carrying large amounts of cholesterol to the arteries.

magnetic resonance imaging (MRI)—A technique for viewing internal organs; an apparatus creating many of the images formerly revealed only by X-rays. MRI uses no radioactive rays.

magnetic therapy—The application of magnets for therapeutic use.

malignant—Dangerous to life; cancerous.

mammogram—A diagnostic X-ray of the breast.

mammography—X-rays of the breast, carried out by special techniques to note the presence or absence of a tumor.

mania—A mental illness characterized by extremes of excitement, happiness, hyperactivity, talkativeness, agitation, grandiosity, and aggression.

manic-depressive—Alternating periods of mania (see above) and depression.

mastectomy—An operation for removal of the breast.

menopause—Change of life; the time of life when a woman's menstrual periods cease.

metabolism—The process by which foods are transformed into basic elements that can be used by the body for energy or growth.

metastasis—The traveling of a disease process from one part of the body to another (e.g., the spread of cancer from its original site).

MRI—See *magnetic resonance imaging.*

myoma—Benign tumor of muscle; also *fibroid.*

myomectomy—Operative removal of a fibroid tumor of the uterus. (The uterus is not removed by this procedure.)

neurosis—An emotional or psychological disorder characterized by anxiety.

nuclear magnetic resonance—See *magnetic resonance imaging.*

oopherectomy—Surgical removal of an ovary. (See also *ovariectomy;* also *castration.*)

osteoporosis—A loss in bony substances producing brittleness and softness of the bones; a condition commonly affecting post-menopausal women and the elderly.

ovariectomy—The surgical removal of the ovaries. See also *castration* and *oopherectomy.*

ovaries—The female gonads, or reproductive glands, on each side of the uterus; their function is to store and release eggs and to manufacture hormones.

ovulation—The process during which the egg is released from the ovary. In normal adult females this occurs once a month.

ovum—An egg; plural is *ova.*

Pap smear—A test used as a screening for cervical cancer; can also detect vaginal cancer.

partial hysterectomy—Also subtotal hysterectomy; the removal of the uterus, but not the cervix.

pectoral muscles—The chest muscles located in the upper chest region.

pelvic inflammatory disease (PID)—A common condition associated with disease of the ovaries and fallopian tubes.

pelvis—The bony ring formed by the bones in the hip region, or pubic bones.

perimenopause—The approximately seven-year transitional period prior to the onset of menopause during which estrogen and progesterone levels begin to decrease.

peri-urethral glands—The aggregate of cells that surround the urethra; the female equivalent to the prostate.

Pfannestiel incision—Also *bikini cut;* a horizontal cut just above the public hairline.

PID—See *pelvic inflammatory disease.*

pituitary gland—An endocrine gland at the base of the brain whose hormones regulate growth.

platelets—*Thrombocytes,* the small colorless discs in circulating blood that aid in blood clotting.

PMS—See *premenstrual syndrome.*

polyp—A growth, usually nonmalignant, of mucous membranes.

postmenopausal bleeding—Bloody vaginal discharge six months or more after a presumed last menstrual period.

precancerous lesion—Tumor tissue that is presently benign but may develop into cancer.

Premarin—The only natural form of estrogen, made from the urine of pregnant horses.

premenstrual syndrome (PMS)—The diagnostic term describing symptoms that occur prior to or around the time of onset of the menstrual flow.

progesterone—The hormone secreted by the ovaries.

prolapsed uterus—See *uterine prolapse.*

prostate—The male gland behind the outlet of the urinary bladder.

puberty—The period of life when the sex organs begin to mature and rapid hormonal changes occur.

pubescence—Adolescence; during puberty, usually between twelve and eighteen years of age.

radiation therapy—The use of X-rays to destroy malignant cells.

radical hysterectomy—Removal of the uterus, cervix, tubes, ovaries, upper vagina, and surrounding connective tissue, performed for a cancerous condition.

rapid plasma reagin (RPR)—Screening test for syphilis.

sarcoma—Malignant tumors developing from connective tissue, bone, or muscle.

serology testing—Studies of the serum of the blood.

serum—That part of whole blood that remains after blood has clotted (yellowish in color).

sexually transmitted disease (STD)—Any disease usually contracted through sexual intimacy; also known as *venereal diseases,* or *VD.*

sonogram—Ultrasound pictures of internal organs.

subtotal hysterectomy—See *partial hysterectomy.*

surgical menopause—The removal of the ovaries; an *oopherectomy* or *castration.* Technically, also refers to the surgical removal of the uterus.

synthetic estrogen—Artificially made compounds that have an estrogenic effect.

testosterone—A hormone that contributes to the development of male characteristics.

thrombophlebitis—Inflammation of a vein with blood clot formation within the vein.

thrombosis—Formation of a blood clot.

total blood cholesterol—The sum of cholesterol carried by the several types of lipoproteins.

total hysterectomy—Also a *complete hysterectomy;* the removal of the uterus, including the cervix.

triglycerides—A fatty acid compound present in everyone; consistently elevated levels of triglycerides may be conductive to premature arteriosclerosis.

tubular pregnancy—See *ectopic pregnancy.*

tumor—A swelling or growth, either cancerous or benign.

ultrasonography—The use of very high frequency sound waves in the visualization of body organs.

ultrasound—See *ultrasonography.*

unopposed HRT—Hormone therapy in which progestin is not included.

urethra—The tube leading from the urinary bladder to the outside.

urinalysis—Examination of the urine.

urinary incontinence—Difficulty in retaining urine.

uterine prolapse—Also *prolapsed uterus.* The abnormal protrusion, or falling, of the uterus through the pelvic floor.

uterine sarcoma—Cancer arising from muscle or fibrous tissue in the wall of the uterus.

uterus—The womb; the female organ in which the embryo develops.

vagina—The female mucous membrane canal leading from the vulva to the cervix of the uterus; the canal in which copulation takes place.

vaginal hernia—Any bulge into the vaginal wall, including uterine prolapse.

Venereal Disease Research Laboratory (VDRL)—Screening test for syphilis, a sexually transmitted disease.

vulva—The external female sex organ composed of the major and minor lips, the clitoris, and the opening of the vagina.

X-ray therapy—Radiation therapy; treatment with X-rays.

X-rays—Light rays of short length that are passed by an electric generator through a glass vacuum tube; electromagnetic radiation that can be used at high levels to treat cancer, and at low levels to diagnose disease.

ZIFT—See *zygote intra fallopian transfer.*

zygote—The fertilization of an egg before it starts to divide and multiply.

zygote intra fallopian transfer (ZIFT)—An assisted reproduction technique; fertilization of the eggs and their initial division into several cells takes place before the eggs are placed into the woman's fallopian tubes, which makes this technique perhaps the most successful.

BIBLIOGRAPHY

BOOKS

Carlson, Karen J., Stephanie A. Eisenstat, and Terra Ziporyn. *The Harvard Guide to Women's Health.* Cambridge, MA: Harvard University Press, 1996.

Curtis, Lindsay R., Glade B. Curtis, and Mary K. Bejard. *My Body—My Decision!* Tucson, AZ: Body Press, 1986.

Cutler, Winnifred. *Hysterectomy: Before and After.* New York: HarperPerennial, 1990.

Foley, Denise, Eileen Nechas, and the editors of *Prevention* Magazine Health Books. *Women's Encyclopedia of Health and Emotional Healing.* New York: Bantam, 1995.

Gifford-Jones, W. *What Every Woman Should Know About Hysterectomy.* Mahwah, NJ: Funk & Wagnalls, 1977.

Giustini, F. G., and F. J. Keefer. *Understanding Hysterectomy: A Woman's Guide.* New York: Walker, 1979.

Gross, Amy, and Dee Ito. *Women Talk About Gynecological Surgery: From Diagnosis to Recovery.* New York: Clarkson Potter, 1991.

Hass, Adelaide, and Susan L. Puretz. *The Women's Guide to Hysterectomy.* Berkeley, CA: Celestial Arts, 1995.

Hite, Shere. *Women and Love.* New York: St. Martin's, 1989.

Huneycutt, Harry C., and Judith L. Davis. *All About Hysterectomy.* Pleasantville, NY: Reader's Digest, 1977.

Jong, Erica. *Fear of Fifty.* New York: HarperPaperbacks, 1994.

Kahn, Ada P., and Linda Hughey Holt. *Midlife Health: A Woman's Practical Guide to Feeling Good.* New York: Avon, 1987.

Kahn, Ada P., and Sheila Kimmel. *Empower Yourself: Every Women's Guide to Self-Esteem.* New York: Avon, 1997.

Masters, William H., Virginia E. Johnson, and Robert C. Kolodny. *Heterosexuality.* New York: HarperPerennial, 1994.

Morgan, Susanne. *Coping with a Hysterectomy.* New York: Dial, 1982.

Northrup, Christiane. *Women's Bodies, Women's Wisdom.* New York: Bantam, 1995.

Nourse, Alan E. *Ladies' Home Journal Family Medical Guide.* New York: Harper & Row, 1973.

Nugent, Nancy. *Hysterectomy: A Complete Up-to-Date Guide to Everything About It and Why It May Be Needed.* New York: Doubleday, 1976.

Rothenberg, Robert E. *The New American Medical Dictionary and Health Manual.* New York: Signet, 1990.

Sachs, Judy. *What Women Can Do About Chronic Endometriosis.* New York: Dell, 1991.

Sheehy, Gail. *Menopause: The Silent Passage.* New York: Pocket Books, 1993.

Stewart, Felicia, Felicia Guest, Gary Stewart, and Robert Hatcher. *Understanding Your Body: Every Woman's Guide to Gynecology and Health.* New York: Bantam, 1987.

Stokes, Naomi Miller. *The Castrated Woman: What Your Doctor Won't Tell You About Hysterectomy.* Danbury, CT: Franklin Watts, 1986.

Stringer, Nelson H. *Uterine Fibroids: What Every Woman Needs to Know.* Glenview, IL: Physicians and Scientists Publishing Co., 1996.

West, Stanley. *The Hysterectomy Hoax.* New York: Doubleday, 1994.

Wison, Robert A. *Feminine Forever.* New York: M. Evans & Co., 1966.

JOURNALS

Alexander, D. A., S. B. Pinion, J. Mollison, H. C. Kitchner, D. E. Parkin, D. R. Abramovich, and I. T. Russell. "Randomized Trial Comparing Hysterectomy with Endometrial Ablation for Dysfunctional Uterine Bleeding." *British Medical Journal* 312, (February 3, 1996):280–284.

Arnot, Bob. "Finding the Right Medical Care Can Mean the Difference Between Life and Death." *Good Housekeeping,* January 1993, p. 58.

Bakos, Susan Crain. "The Operation I Didn't Have." *Ladies Home Journal,* November 1993, p. 100.

Bernhard, L. A. "Consequences of Hysterectomy in the Lives of Women." *Health Care for Women International* 13, no. 3 (July–September 1992):281–291.

Bernhard, L. A. "Men's Views About Hysterectomies and Women Who Have Them." *Image: The Journal of Nursing Scholarship* 24, no. 3 (Fall 1992):177–181.

Carlson, Karen J., David H. Nichols, and Isaac Schiff. "Indications for Hysterectomy." *New England Journal of Medicine* 328, no. 12 (March 25, 1993):856.

Chapple, A. "Hysterectomy: British National Health Service and Private Patients Have Very Different Experiences." *Journal of Advanced Nursing* 22, no. 5 (November 1995):900–906.

Cohen, S. M., A. O. Hollingsworth, and M. Rubin. "Another Look at Psychological Complications of Hysterectomy." *Image: The Journal of Nursing Scholarship* 21, no. 1 (Spring 1989):51–53.

Dorsey, James H., and David A. Grimes. "Technology Follies: Curtain Call." *Journal of the American Medical Association,* no. 19 (November 17, 1993):2298.

Dranov, Paula. "When the Diagnosis Is Fibroids: New Treatments Will Prevent Hysterectomy for Millions of Women." *American Health* 12, no. 7 (September 1993):68.

Dresher, Olivia. "I've Lost My Essence." *Menopause News* 6, no. 4 (July–August 1996):3.

Dwyer, James, Nina Cerfolio, Thomas H. Murray, and Miriam B. Rosenthal. "The Value of a Uterus." *Hastings Center Report* 26, no. 2 (March–April 1996):28.

Everson, S. A., K. A. Matthews, D. S. Guzick, R. R. Wing, and L. H. Kuller. "Effects of Surgical Menopause on Psychological Characteristics and Lipid Levels: The Healthy Women Study." *Health Psychology* 14, no. 5 (September 1995):435–443.

Federkow, Donna M., and Richard E. Kalbfleisch. "Total Abdominal Hysterectomy at Abdominal Sacrovaginopexy: A Comparative Study." *American Journal of Obstetrics and Gynecology* 169, no. 3 (September 1993):641.

Filiberti, A., M. Regazzoni, M. Garavoglia, C. Perilli, P. Alpinelli, G. Santoni, A. Attili, and B. Stefanon. "Problems After Hysterectomy: A Comparative Content Analysis of 60 Interviews with Cancer and Non-cancer Hysterectomized Women." *European Journal of Gynaecological Oncology* 12, no. 6 (1991):445–449.

Friedman, Andrew J., and Susan T. Haas. "Should Uterine Size Be an Indication for Surgical Intervention in Women with Myomas?" *American Journal of Obstetrics and Gynecology* 168, no. 3 (March 1993):751.

Gath, D., N. Rose, A. Bond, A. Day, A. Garrod, and S. Hodges. "Hysterectomy and Psychiatric Disorder: Are the Levels of

Psychiatric Morbidity Falling?" *Psychological Medicine* 25, no. 2 (March 1995):277–283.

Geller, Stacie E., Lawton R. Burns, and David J. Brailer. "The Impact of Nonclinical Factors on Practice Variations: The Case of Hysterectomies." *Health Services Research* 30, no. 6 (February 1996): 729.

Grimes, David A. "Primary Prevention of Ovarian Cancer." *Journal of the American Medical Association* 270, no. 23 (December 15, 1993):2855.

Grimes, David A. "Shifting Indications for Hysterectomy: Nature, Nurture, or Neither?" *Lancet* 344, no. 8938 (December 17, 1994): 1652.

Helstrom, L. "Sexuality After Hysterectomy: A Model Based on Quantitative Analysis of 104 Women Before and After Subtotal Hysterectomy." *Journal of Psychosomatic Obstetrics and Gynecology* 15, no. 4 (December 1994):219–229.

Helstrom, L., P. O. Lundberg, D. Sorbom, and T. Backstrom. "Sexuality After Hysterectomy: A Factor Analysis of Women's Sexual Lives Before and After Subtotal Hysterectomy." *Obstetrics and Gynecology* 81, (March 1993):357–362.

"Hysterectomy and Its Alternatives: One Small Step Toward Assessing the Options." *HealthFacts* 19, no. 180 (May 1994):3.

"Hysterectomy Hesitation." *Harvard Health Letter* 19, no. 2 (December 1993):8.

Kilkku, P., V. Lehtinen, T. Hirvonen, and M. Gronroos. "Abdominal Hysterectomy Versus Supravaginal Uterine Amputation: Psychic Factors." *Annales Chirurgiac et Gynaccologiac (Suppl.)* 202 (1987):62–67.

Kinnick, V., and D. Leners. "The Hysterectomy Experience: An Ethnographic Study." *Journal of Holistic Nursing* 13, no. 2 (June 1995):142–154.

Lalinee-Michaud, M., and F. Engelsmann. "Cultural Factors and Reaction to Hysterectomy." *Social Psychiatry and Psychiatric Epidemiology* 24 (May 1989):165–171.

Liu, W. H., P. J. Standen, and A. R. Aitkenhead. "Therapeutic Suggestions During General Anaesthesia in Patients Undergoing Hysterectomy." *British Journal of Anesthesia* 68, no. 3 (March 1992): 277–281.

Metcalf, M. G., J. H. Livesey, J. E. Wells, V. Braiden, S. M. Hudson, and L. Bamber. "Premenstrual Syndrome in Hysterectomized Women: Mood and Physical Symptom Cyclicity." *Journal of Psychosomatic Research* 35, nos. 4–5 (1991):555–567.

Mwaba, K., and E. B. Lotloenyano. "Attitudes and Knowledge About Hysterectomy: A Study of Women in Mmabtho." *Curationis* 17, no. 3 (August 1994):2–3.

Myers, Evan R., Ann-Louise S. Silver, Chris Wahlberg, S. Elizabeth Whitmore, Steven Lehrer, Susan E. Hankinson, David J. Hunter, Graham A. Colditz, and Frank E. Speizer. "Tubal Ligation, Hysterectomy, and Risk of Ovarian Cancer." *Journal of the American Medical Association* 27, no. 16 (April 27, 1994):1235.

Nathorst-Boos, J., T. Fuchs, and B. von Schoultz. "Consumer's Attitude to Hysterectomy: The Experience of 678 Women." *Acta Obstetrica et Gynecologica Scandinavica,* no. 3 (April 1992):230–234.

Nathorst-Boos, J., and B. von Schoultz. "Psychological Reactions and Sexual Life After Hysterectomy with and Without Ophorectomy." *Gynecologic and Obstetric Investigation* 34, no. 2 (1992):97–101.

Nathorst-Boos, J., B. von Schoultz, and K. Carlstrom. "Elective Ovarian Removal and Estrogen Replacement Therapy—Effects of Sexual life, Psychological Well-being and Androgen Status." *Journal of Psychosomatic Obstetrics and Gynecology* 14, no. 4 (December 1993):283–293.

Oldenhave, Anna, Lazlo J. B. Jaszmann, Walter T. A. M. Everaerd, and Ary A. Haspels. "Hysterectomized Women with Ovarian Conservation Report More Severe Climacteric Complaints Than Do Normal Climacteric Women of Similar Age." *American Journal of Obstetrics and Gynecology* 168, no. 3 (March 1993):765.

Osborne, M. F., and D. H. Gath. "Psychological and Physical Determinants of Premenstrual Symptoms Before and After Hysterectomy." *Psychological Medicine* 20, no. 3 (August 1990):565–572.

Payer, Lynn. "The Operation Every Woman Should Question." *McCall's,* June 1995, p. 54.

Ryan, M. M., L. Dennerstein, and R. Pepperell. "Psychological Aspects of Hysterectomy: A Prospective Study." *British Journal of Psychiatry* 154 (April 1989):516–522.

Schofield, M. J., A. Bennett, S. Redman, W. A. Walters, and R. W. Sanson-Fisher. "Self-Reported Longterm Outcomes of Hysterectomy." *British Journal of Obstetrics and Gynaecology* 98, no. 11 (November 1991):1129–1136.

Thomas, V., M. Heath, D. Rose, and P. Flory. "Psychological Characteristics and the Effectiveness of Patient Controlled Analgesia." *British Journal of Anesthesia* 74, no. 3 (March 1995):271–276.

Webb, C. "Professional and Lay Social Support for Hysterectomy Patients." *Journal of Advanced Nursing* 11, no. 2 (March 1986): 167–177.

Williams, P. D., D. M. Valderrama, M. D. Gloria, L. G. Pascoguin, I. D. Saavedra, D. T. De la Rama, T. C. Fetty, C. M. Abaguin, and S. B. Zaldivar. "Effects of Preparation of Mastectomy/Hysterectomy on Women's Post-operative Self-Care Behaviors." *International Journal of Nursing Studies* 25, no. 3 (1988):191–206.

Williamson, M. L. "Sexual Adjustment After Hysterectomy." *Journal of Obstetric, Gynecologic, and Neonatal Nursing* 21, no. 1 (January–February 1992):42–47.

INDEX

F

G

T

U

V

W

Y

Z